Copyright and Use of This Book

For information contact RefluxMD by emailing refluxdiet@refluxmd.com.

Edited by: Allison M. Sidhu
Cover design by: Vanessa Maynard
Cover photo: iStockphoto

FIRST EDITION
Prepared by RefluxMD
June 1, 2015

D1482211

Preface

There is a worldwide epidemic today, and it is not whooping cough or measles as you may have been led to expect by listening to today's news. Gastroesophageal reflux disease (GERD), also known as acid reflux, is widespread, chronic and rapidly expanding throughout the world.

Consider these statistics:

- Over 85 million adults in the US experience GERD symptoms monthly.

- 45 to 50 million of these suffer several times each week.

- An additional 100 million in western Europe, Australia, New Zealand and Japan have symptoms monthly, with 46 million suffering weekly.

- Prevalence of esophageal cancer, resulting directly from GERD, has increased over 600% since 1975, making this disease the fastest growing type of cancer in the US.

Very few adults are aware of these statistics. When talking with an old colleague of mine about why this disease has so little visibility today, he looked at me and asked, "No one ever died from heartburn, right?" WRONG! This year, over 20,000 deaths due to adenocarcinoma of the esophagus are anticipated, most of which will be exclusively attributed to GERD.

Working closely with several of the top GERD physicians in the US, we launched RefluxMD to raise awareness, to bring accurate and honest information to sufferers, and to help them build a path to relief and good health. Our medical advisors recommended a particular strategy to find relief as an alternative to the current "status quo" treatment plan – long-term daily use of proton pump inhibitors. This model has six elements that every GERD sufferer should seriously consider:

1. Partnering with a GERD medical expert rather than your family doctor

2. Managing your weight to maintain a healthy level

3. Modifying your diet to eat healthy foods and avoid trigger foods

4. Making lifestyle changes to reduce symptoms

5. Using the least powerful anti-reflux medications to achieve symptom relief

6. Considering anti-reflux surgery if satisfactory symptom relief is not achieved

Since its founding, RefluxMD has addressed all of the topics listed above via articles and stories on its website, as well as online tools. We have connected thousands of our members and website visitors with GERD experts across the country. However, RefluxMD was unable to provide the highest quality support in two areas – weight management and diet modifications. Unfortunately, we found ourselves unhappy with the extent of our ability to help our members manage their weight at a healthy level, as well as our ability to provide guidance for a healthy and GERD-friendly eating plan.

Do we need another eating and dieting program?

Initially, we did not think so. Our goal was to find a high-quality diet program and promote it as part of RefluxMD's solution package. After looking at many of the existing online diet programs and books, we were surprised and saddened that no comprehensive and high-quality GERD-friendly resource was available. Our only option was to build our own.

RefluxMD's Eating Plan and Diet Program was built from the ground up. It is based on the #1 diet program today, the DASH Diet, and utilizes the knowledge of top experts in medicine, nutrition, and psychology. Section I provides all of the information required to understand GERD – its causes, symptoms, treatments and procedures. Sections II and III discuss nutrition, diet and RefluxMD's approach to GERD-friendly eating and weight loss. Section IV focuses on the psychological aspects of making such a life change, and offers keys to weight loss success. Finally, Sections V and VI provide daily meal plans and recipes to help you to get started on the program.

This book was written for you and all individuals who struggle with GERD. You can reclaim control of your life and find relief, but you must make changes first, and change can be difficult. Take your time as you read through this program. Avoid the impulse to jump right in to the daily meal plans and recipes. Relief will come with a greater understanding of this disease, nutrition, and the mental aspects necessary for success.

Finally, we want to thank all of those who helped RefluxMD reach hundreds of thousands of GERD sufferers, and those who assisted with the creation of this diet program. First, our thanks go to our medical advisors, who helped us to understand this disease and all of the treatment alternatives – Senior Advisor Tom DeMeester, MD; Medical Director William Dengler, MD; and Scientific Director Para Chandrasoma, MD.

We sincerely want to thank the many outside contributors to this book for their help and assistance. It was a pleasure working with all of you to develop this unique and innovative dietary approach to acid reflux disease.

Michael R. Edelstein, Ph.D.
Practicing psychologist, published author and lecturer
San Francisco, CA

Dr. Michael R. Edelstein is a practicing psychologist (in person, Skype, and via telephone therapy) in the San Francisco Bay Area who specializes in the treatment of anxiety, depression, relationship problems and addictions. He is the author of Three Minute Therapy, a self-help book for overcoming common emotional and behavioral problems, for which he was awarded Author of the Year. Throughout his career, Dr. Edelstein has utilized Rational Emotive Behavior Therapy (REBT) approach to assist adults in making and mastering behavioral lifestyle changes, in pursuit of a happier life. With the simple yet powerful tools that he has created, Dr. Edelstein has successfully taught thousands of adults how to face difficulties in their lives and make lasting changes in the way they think, act, and feel. Other books published by Dr. Edelstein are Stage Fright, which includes interviews with Robin Williams, Jason Alexander, Melissa Etheridge, Maya Angelou and others, relating their personal experiences and wisdom in coping with performance anxiety; Rational Drinking: How to Live Happily With or Without Alcohol, which presents concepts, tools and strategies for overcoming compulsive drinking; and Therapy Breakthrough (with David Ramsey Steele and Richard Kujoth), a history and critique of the psychotherapy movement from Sigmund Freud to Albert Ellis. Dr. Edelstein was a training supervisor and fellow of the Albert Ellis Institute. He holds a diplomate in cognitive-behavioral therapy from the National Association of Cognitive-Behavioral Therapists, and is on its board of advisors. He was president of the Association for Behavioral and Cognitive Therapy. He is a certified sex therapist and has served as a consulting psychologist for the National Save-A-Life League, Inc., the oldest suicide prevention center in the United States. Dr. Edelstein was also a professional advisor to the San Francisco SMART Recovery Program. He was trained in REBT by Albert Ellis.

David S. Johnson, MD, FACS
Premier Surgical Associates
Palm Springs, CA

Dr. David Johnson founded Premier Surgical Associates in Palm Springs, California to serve patients in the Coachella Valley. He is currently establishing a treatment center with a local hospital to treat GERD, as well as other esophageal and foregut disorders. Dr. Johnson became active with RefluxMD during its first year in 2012, offering his medical perspective and developing content to share with members. He holds a Bachelor of Arts degree in biology, graduating magna cum laude from Boston University. He also holds a Doctorate of Medicine from the John A. Burns School of Medicine at the University of Hawaii in Honolulu. He continued his training with a Categorical Surgical Internship and Surgical Residency at the University of Hawaii

Surgical Residency Program in Honolulu, where he was selected to be Chief Resident in Surgery. Board certified by the American Board of Surgery, Dr. Johnson settled in California in 2009. He maintains privileges at Hemet Valley Medical Center, Menifee Valley Medical Center, Inland Valley Medical Center, Corona Regional Medical Center, Desert Regional Medical Center, Eisenhower Medical Center, JFK Memorial Hospital, and Loma Linda Medical Center, Murrieta. Dr. Johnson is a fellow of the American College of Surgeons and an active member of the American Medical Association and Riverside County Medical Association. Dr. Johnson is the author of numerous articles and abstracts that have been published in peer-reviewed journals. In addition, Dr. Johnson has given lectures at various surgical conferences and meetings around the country and has an appointment as an Assistant Clinical Professor with UC Riverside.

Kimberly A. Tessmer RDN, LD
Consulting dietitian, nutritionist, and published author
Founder, Nutrition Focus

Kimberly Tessmer is a Registered Dietitian Nutritionist and Licensed Dietitian in the State of Ohio as well as a published author. She is the founder and owner of Nutrition Focus, which offers a wide range of nutritional services for individuals online as well as both small and large organizations and businesses. Ms. Tessmer has over twenty years of experience in the field of nutrition and has authored nine books to date with more to come. She holds a Bachelor of Science degree in technology and dietetics from Bowling Green State University in Bowling Green, Ohio. Ms. Tessmer has extensive experience in this area. She worked in hospitals, nursing homes, and as a corporate dietitian for three national weight loss companies before launching Nutrition Focus. You can connect with Ms. Tessmer via Facebook and Twitter, and her books can be purchased from Amazon in various formats.

Are you ready to get started?

OK, are you ready to find your path to relief and good health? Our experts believe that what you learn in this program will enable you to make positive changes in your life, so let us get started! From all of us at RefluxMD and those who have already participated in this diet program, we sincerely wish you the best as you seek the relief that you deserve!

Sincerely,
Bruce Kaechele
RefluxMD Founder

Table of Contents

Section I
GERD: The Disease

Introduction
Message from Dr. David S. Johnson, MD, FACS, GERD Expert and Surgeon

"I believe the most important factor in this disease is YOU. YOU have the means to manage your symptoms. YOU are the most important factor impacting the progression of your disease."

As a GERD expert and anti-reflux surgeon, I am constantly frustrated by how little most adults know about gastroesophageal reflux disease, better known as GERD or acid reflux. It is estimated that one in three adults experience GERD symptoms at least once a month, and one in five experience symptoms every week. Driving my frustration is the fact that most of my patients could have avoided their first visit to my office, had they taken their symptoms more seriously earlier.

When RefluxMD asked me to write the introduction to Section I of this book, I saw it as an opportunity to reach many adults who are suffering from GERD and to offer valuable information about this chronic condition. It is through increased awareness and knowledge that GERD sufferers can make effective decisions with their physicians to properly treat their disease.

For many in the early stages of GERD, a focus on weight management, diet, lifestyle choices, and the proper use of anti-reflux medications can not only reduce or eliminate the symptoms, it can actually stop or slow the potential progression of their disease. Unfortunately, as this disease progresses, these elements of treatment have less of an impact on disease progression. More powerful medications and procedural interventions may be required to avoid serious complications.

I believe the most important factor in this disease is YOU. YOU have the means to manage your symptoms. YOU are the most important factor impacting the progression of your disease. YOU have many treatment options that can provide relief and improve the quality of your life – and it is up to YOU to make these critical decisions.

Section I of this book will help you to make important decisions about treating your disease. RefluxMD has taken a complicated long-term chronic condition and made it simple for individuals who are not medical professionals to understand. This section lays the foundation that you will need to make personal decisions with the guidance of your physician, as you take more responsibility for managing your disease. This section of the book will cover many important topics including:

- Information necessary to understand your long-term chronic condition and how to build a plan to manage your disease.

- The negative aspects of today's "status quo" treatment model that have led to a dramatic increase in the incidence of Barrett's esophagus, a precancerous condition, and adenocarcinoma, or reflux-induced esophageal cancer.

- The underlying causes of reflux disease and the related symptoms.

- The honest facts about anti-reflux medication, enabling you to determine for yourself the necessity of powerful prescription or over the counter (OTC) drugs.

- A thorough explanation of treatment options including lifestyle changes, home remedies, medications and surgeries.

- Ways to develop a plan to gain relief from symptoms and improved health.

- The importance of a team to ensure success as you design your plan and travel your path to health.

This section is designed to be a general broad overview of GERD rather than a deep dive into understanding the disease. The chapters in this section are based upon the principles and clinical experience of RefluxMD's medical advisors and GERD experts across the country. You may have more questions after reviewing this information. I encourage you to visit RefluxMD's website for more detailed answers to your questions. I also suggest that you take your questions to a GERD expert who may be found using RefluxMD's Find-a-Physician tool.

Finally, I encourage you to learn all you can about your disease, because it is YOUR disease, and it is also YOUR responsibility to manage your disease. As a GERD expert, I am here to help you to understand all of your options and to assist you in making decisions about your medical treatment. In the end, that decision is yours and yours alone. I hope this book will lead you to a better understanding of GERD and down a new path towards relief and good health.

Sincerely,
Dr. David Johnson

About Dr. David Johnson

Dr. David Johnson founded Premier Surgical Associates in Palm Springs, California to serve patients in the Coachella Valley. He is currently establishing a treatment center with a local hospital to treat GERD, as well as other esophageal and foregut disorders. Dr. Johnson became active with RefluxMD during its first year in 2012, offering his medical perspective and developing content to share with members. He holds a Bachelor of Arts degree in biology, graduating magna cum laude from Boston University. He also holds a Doctorate of Medicine from the John A. Burns School of Medicine at the University of Hawaii in Honolulu. He continued his training with a Categorical Surgical Internship and Surgical Residency at the University of Hawaii Surgical Residency Program in Honolulu, where he was selected to be Chief Resident in Surgery. Board certified by the American Board of Surgery, Dr. Johnson settled in California in 2009. He maintains privileges at Hemet Valley Medical Center, Menifee Valley Medical Center, Inland Valley Medical Center, Corona Regional Medical Center, Desert Regional Medical Center, Eisenhower Medical Center, JFK Memorial Hospital, and Loma Linda Medical Center, Murrieta. Dr. Johnson is a fellow of the American College of Surgeons and an active member of the American Medical Association and Riverside County Medical Association. Dr. Johnson is the author of numerous articles and abstracts that have been published in peer-reviewed journals. In addition, Dr. Johnson has given lectures at various surgical conferences and meetings around the country and has an appointment as an Assistant Clinical Professor with UC Riverside.

Section I: Overview

*"Far too many people continue to struggle with the painful symptoms of GERD because they do not think there is anything they can do. **But that is just not true.**"*

Laying the Foundation

So you have GERD. You are not alone. In fact, almost a third of adults experience the symptoms of GERD on a monthly basis, which is remarkable when you consider how little media attention this growing epidemic currently receives. Perhaps this condition is often dismissed as a nuisance BECAUSE it affects so many people, despite the fact that sufferers experience significant physical, emotional and economic impacts. Although the medical community continues to develop more effective drugs to alleviate the symptoms of reflux disease, the rate and severity of the disease as well as the frequency of complications continue to grow. Medical experts view reflux disease as an epidemic, yet little is being done to improve our ability to manage it. We believe that needs to change.

And that change begins with you.

The most important point we can stress is that **you should not have to suffer** just because you have GERD. Far too many people continue to struggle with the painful symptoms of GERD because they do not think there is anything they can do. But that is just not true. Following a GERD-friendly diet is a critical first step on the path to relief and is often the first recommendation that GERD experts give their patients. The goal of the RefluxMD diet plan is to give you the tools that you need to take control of your health and FEEL BETTER!

Section I of this book lays the foundation for putting the RefluxMD GERD Diet Plan into action. Learning about your disease – its most common symptoms, how it occurs, why it often progresses, and how it is diagnosed and treated – will help you to understand why diet is such a critical piece of the treatment puzzle.

Chapter 1 - GERD: A Growing Epidemic
Chapter 2 - The GERD Patient Bill of Rights
Chapter 3 - The Underlying Causes of GERD
Chapter 4 - The Symptoms that Indicate GERD
Chapter 5 - The Stages of GERD: Why You Need to Know Yours
Chapter 6 - Complications if GERD is not Treated Properly
Chapter 7 - The Importance of Diagnostic Testing
Chapter 8 - Lifestyle Choices to Treat GERD
Chapter 9 - Using Medications to Treat GERD
Chapter 10 - Surgical Alternatives for GERD Treatment
Chapter 11 - Home Remedies to Manage Your Symptoms

Chapter 1
GERD: A Growing Epidemic

"GERD is not just a nuisance. It is a long-term chronic condition that can progress if not managed properly."

How Many People Have GERD?

Do you consider a disease that affects between twenty and thirty-three percent of all adults an epidemic? Would you expect national health agencies to respond with an all-out effort to slow and ultimately stop the growth of a disease that impacts so many? While we have seen this level of response to many illnesses in the past – such as typhoid, polio, measles, whooping cough, etc. – this has not been the case with gastroesophageal reflux disease, also known as GERD or acid reflux. Let us look at some of the facts about GERD:

- 75 million American adults, or 1 in 3, have symptoms monthly, and 50 million American adults, or 1 in 5, have symptoms weekly.

- Over the counter (OTC) and prescription medications to treat acid reflux cost Americans over $10 billion annually.

- The average annual medical costs for an individual with GERD are $3,355 higher than expenses for an individual without GERD.

- GERD costs employers an estimated $1.9 billion a week due to lost productivity and chronic absences. That is almost $100 billion annually.

- The incidence of GERD in American adults is increasing at a rate of 30% every decade since the 1970s.

GERD is not just a problem in the United States. There are an estimated 190 million adults suffering from acid reflux disease today when we include Canada, Europe, Japan, and Australia. These 190 million are not just experiencing minor discomfort – their experiences are generally much worse than that. For more than half of sufferers, GERD seriously impacts their quality of life. Many miss work, they cancel social plans with friends and family, they cannot go out to dinner, and some are forced to sleep in a chair since they cannot lie flat in bed. GERD is not just a nuisance; it is a long-term chronic condition that can progress if it is not managed properly.

Why has nothing been done?

The general attitude of most adults with GERD is that acid reflux is just a nuisance. In fact, during the early stages of reflux disease, it is rare to find anyone who takes their symptoms seriously. Each year, heartburn sends over 200,000 adults rushing to the emergency room for a presumed heart attack. Most of those 200,000 choose not to recognize their earlier, less severe symptoms as a disease. They simply ignore the important messages their body is sending them, only to be awakened later when a heart attack scare alarms them into taking real action.

Here are some of the most frequent excuses for ignoring GERD symptoms:

It is just my food choices.

It is amazing how little most people know about reflux disease. Many still think it is all about the pepperoni pizza or the spicy hot sauce they ate last night. In reality, GERD symptoms are caused by a structural weakness in the esophagus. The lower esophageal sphincter (LES), located at the junction of the esophagus and the stomach, performs an important function similar to that of a valve. When working properly, it creates a very effective barrier between the esophagus and the stomach. However, when the LES loses its barrier function, stomach contents can move freely up into the esophagus. As a result, the stomach acids that typically remain in the stomach can reach the esophagus, creating pain and often doing serious damage.

My pills cured me.

Proton pump inhibitor medications (PPIs) such as Nexium and Prilosec do not cure GERD; they only control symptoms for some people. One of the biggest problems with how GERD is currently treated is that physicians often prescribe long-term daily PPIs without explaining what they can and cannot do. Patients may take these drugs for years without ever understanding that PPIs only mask the symptoms of their disease. Though the pain may subside, the reflux continues and their disease may progress.

I just love my lifestyle and I cannot give up certain things.

Another problem with simply managing the symptoms of GERD with PPIs is that they enable the exact lifestyle that, in many cases, created the disease. Without these medications, most sufferers would be forced to make dietary and lifestyle changes to avoid the painful symptoms of heartburn. Since PPIs can be so effective at controlling symptoms, the bad habits continue, leaving the door open to potential disease progression.

It is just about excess acid in the stomach.

This could not be further from the truth. Everyone has a significant amount of stomach acid, whether they suffer from GERD or not. Since antacids and PPIs reduce the acidity of the stomach, most people just assume that they "make too much" acid. This is generally false, since the stomach was designed to have a high acid level to promote good digestion.

Five Facts You Need to Know About GERD

1. Reflux is a long-term chronic condition that can progress if left untreated.

Heartburn is just a result of what we eat, right? Wrong!

As noted earlier, reflux disease is caused by a weak LES, the ring of muscle located in the lower end of the esophagus. Reflux can happen for a variety of reasons: eating large portions, obesity, smoking, and excessive consumption of alcohol are all known to damage or weaken the LES. Over time, the longer you indulge in these activities, the more you potentially weaken the LES. Because the lining of the esophagus is easily irritated by the contents of the stomach, reflux disease can lead to complications such as inflammation, erosions of the lining of the esophagus, narrowing of the esophagus, Barrett's esophagus (a precancerous condition) and esophageal cancer.

2. Reflux disease is directly linked to esophageal cancer.

No one ever died from heartburn, right? Wrong!

Esophageal adenocarcinoma, a type of cancer of the esophagus, is directly linked to reflux disease. In fact, reflux disease is the only known cause for this type of cancer. The number of esophageal cancer cases has grown over 600% since 1975, making this deadly disease the fastest growing type of cancer in the United States. When charted against the incidence of all other cancers, esophageal cancer is in a league of its own. Sadly, esophageal adenocarcinoma is also one of the most lethal types of cancer. The overall likelihood of surviving five years beyond a diagnosis is only fifteen to seventeen percent. In 2015 alone, it is predicted that approximately 20,000 deaths will result from reflux-induced esophageal cancer.

3. Today's "status quo" treatment for GERD has serious limitations and risks.

OTC and prescription medications stop the reflux, right? Wrong!

Many times, when a patient complains of the symptoms of reflux, a PPI such as Prilosec, Prevacid, or Nexium is prescribed by a physician or is simply purchased over the counter at a drugstore. These drugs relieve the symptoms of reflux by reducing the amount of acid produced by the stomach, which helps to minimize or even eliminate heartburn symptoms. Unfortunately, reducing heartburn does not mean the reflux is cured. Taking PPIs does not stop the reflux, it only stops the heartburn and the disease continues to progress.

4. There are potential negative side effects associated with daily PPI use.

Those PPIs must be safe since they are sold over the counter and do not need a doctor's prescription, right? Wrong!

Consumers spend more than $20 billion worldwide each year on PPIs (over $10 billion in the U.S. annually), looking for relief from their reflux symptoms. While these medications have helped millions of people, there are potential risks associated with them that users must understand. Reflux disease is a chronic progressive disease. Once PPIs are started, use typically continues on a daily basis indefinitely. Studies have shown that long-term daily use of these drugs is associated with an increase in the incidence of bone fractures, *Clostridium difficile* colitis (a potentially deadly infection of the intestines), pneumonia and low magnesium levels. PPIs are also known to interact with other drugs. The most notable of these is Plavix, a blood thinner used for the prevention of heart attacks and strokes. It is most distressing to note that several studies have documented that thirty percent of PPI users do not even have reflux. This means millions of people are taking these drugs unnecessarily.

5. You can manage your reflux disease!
There must be something that can be done to stop symptoms and the progression of reflux disease, right? RIGHT!

Although reflux disease cannot be reversed, the good news is that most people with reflux can effectively manage their symptoms and impact the progression of their disease. These options change as the disease progresses, so getting an early start is important.

Get Started Today

An actual GERD-sufferer's account of her experience might help the five facts described above to hit closer to home. We are confident that this woman would have done things differently had she been aware of the facts of her disease earlier in her life:

> *"By the time the paramedics got to me I thought I was dying of a heart attack, so imagine my relief when I found out it was only heartburn. When the doctor sent me home with a prescription, I had not a care in the world, so confident was I that the prescribed medicine would cure me. And I thought it did because I felt fine and could eat just about anything I wanted for a long time. It was like a miracle until eventually, after years of taking PPIs daily, my symptoms came back with a vengeance. No amount of medicine stopped the pain. Desperate for help, I sought the care of a specialist and was shocked to be diagnosed with esophageal cancer. After several weeks of chemotherapy, surgeons removed my esophagus and gave me the devastating news that the cancer had spread to my lymph nodes. While I am determined to keep fighting, the anger and frustration that I feel is overwhelming. Why was I not warned that my heartburn symptoms were only being masked by the medication I was taking? Why was I not told about the possibility that my disease could be progressing like a silent killer to a deadly stage? I am fifty-two years old, a*

wife and a mother of three, and I just want to live."
If you have reflux disease, then this resource is for you. There is a lot to do! First, educate yourself about this chronic condition and know where you are in the progression of your disease. Then, take steps to stop that progression, monitor your symptoms, design a personal reflux disease management plan, and build a team of family, friends and medical professionals who can help you on your journey to good health.

Chapter 2
The GERD Patient Bill of Rights

"The current medical approach to reflux disease is a path to massive financial costs and increased suffering."

The "Status Quo" Treatment Model

In January 2012, a group of top GERD physicians spent several days together in Pasadena, California to discuss why the incidence of reflux disease was growing unchecked and to determine what, if anything, could be done about it. It was clear that the "status quo" treatment plan used by most physicians was not working. In most respects, incidence of the disease continues to increase every year. Several facts were evident:

1. Primary care physicians (PCPs) are not adequately trained to diagnose or treat GERD. It is estimated that less than thirty percent of all physician visits where GERD was the primary diagnosis were with specialists who have the equipment and training to diagnose GERD accurately. Consequently, diagnoses for the remaining seventy percent were done via "symptom reporting" with PCP treatment, which has led to an overall gross misdiagnosis of GERD. Consequently, this widespread misdiagnosis has led to an over-prescription of PPI medication. It is estimated that over thirty percent of all PPI users should not be on this medication.

2. Most of the specialists who accurately diagnose GERD recommend the same treatment protocol as primary care physicians – daily PPI usage. In most cases, this becomes a prescription for life. If symptoms return, the recommendation is typically to double the medication dosage. Unfortunately, it is rare for those prescribing physicians to disclose these important facts to their patients about the treatment plan: 1. PPI medications only treat symptoms and are not a cure for reflux disease; 2. the disease may still continue to progress while using PPIs, even when symptoms are absent; 3. long-term daily use of PPIs has several potential negative side effects, as documented on the FDA-mandated packaging inserts; and 4. there are alternative treatments that should be considered by all patients with GERD.

3. Medical societies and associations have demonstrated little or no interest in challenging the "status quo" treatment model.

4. The big winners are the pharmaceutical manufacturers who have spent millions in advertising dollars to promote their medications directly to

GERD sufferers.

5. The American healthcare system spends $3 billion annually on anti-reflux medications for individuals who do not have reflux disease.

6. The biggest losers are those GERD sufferers who are put on the "status quo" treatment plan, believing they have cured their disease but developing serious complications years later with a deteriorating quality of life.

The Pasadena Protocol

The Pasadena Protocol was developed as a response to the current "status quo" method of diagnosing and treating reflux disease. The Pasadena Protocol is a set of conventions, principles and behaviors that have the power to dramatically impact relationships between patients, practitioners, insurers and employers. The Pasadena Protocol is a powerful tool to achieve the following objectives:

- Improved long-term medical outcomes for the treatment of reflux disease.

- Enhanced quality of life for patients suffering from reflux disease.

- Lower healthcare costs associated with the treatment of reflux disease.

Every physician should not only agree with these principles, but should also actively follow them. For patients, this is their Bill of Rights.

Elements of the Pasadena Protocol

1. Educated and empowered patients are essential to success.

2. Reflux disease sufferers deserve an assessment of their disease along with relevant recommendations.

3. Knowledgeable GERD experts should treat those with reflux disease.

4. Powerful anti-reflux medications must be prescribed appropriately.

5. A support team is essential to successfully managing reflux disease.

6. Reflux disease is a progressive chronic condition that requires long-term monitoring.

7. The reflux community must be informed and responsive as new technologies, knowledge and treatments become available.

Changing the Future of Reflux Disease

The "status quo" treatment model is failing and must change. We should not have to hear even one more story like this:

"I am a sixty-eight-year-old white male who has suffered from acid reflux for most of my adult life. About fifteen years ago, I was placed on Prilosec by my gastro doc. After that, I had few symptoms of reflux and heartburn. Since I had no significant symptoms, neither my primary care doc nor my gastro doc ever recommended an endoscopy. I never thought about asking for one since I thought symptom control meant reflux control and healing. Then, about two years ago when all the scares started coming out about long-term use of PPIs and since I was having no significant symptoms of reflux, I asked my primary care doc if I could stop the Prilosec to see if symptoms returned. My symptoms did not change and that affirmed my belief that the Prilosec had allowed my esophagus to heal.

Then, about a year after going off the Prilosec I was diagnosed with stage 3 esophageal adenocarcinoma. Since then, until I found RefluxMD, I beat up on myself and blamed myself for going off the Prilosec, believing this was the cause of the cancer. My gastro doc clearly thought this was what caused the cancer, although my oncologist said being off the medication for only a year was not enough time to allow the cancer to develop. I now think both doctors are wrong in their reasoning. What I have read at RefluxMD indicates to me that going off the Prilosec did not cause the cancer, nor did stopping the drug "cold turkey" (which I later read could result in serious damage to the esophagus due to "rebound reflux"), since all the Prilosec was doing was controlling the symptoms for all those years rather than stopping the progression of disease.

Although knowing the answer to this question will not change the fact that I have cancer or the probable outcome, it is important to me to feel that I did not operate in an irresponsible way concerning my healthcare, based on the best information and medical guidance available to me at the time. I also want to share information with friends and family who are taking these drugs, and I want what I tell them to be accurate."

Although the incidence of cancer is still relatively small, with eighteen thousand projected deaths this year, that number is still increasing despite billions spent on today's "status quo" medication therapy. The current medical approach may reduce short-term symptoms for some, but research suggests it will result in a higher rate of disease progression for many, leading to an increased incidence of esophagitis, Barrett's esophagus, and esophageal adenocarcinoma. Additionally, improper and unnecessary treatment adds a tremendous financial burden to the healthcare system. The Pasadena Protocol is a response to this possible future. Comprised of the principles and concepts noted above, this new outlook has the potential to change the behavior toward reflux disease and address the severe shortcomings of today's treatment model.

Chapter 3
The Underlying Causes of GERD

"GERD occurs when the valve between the stomach and the esophagus is unable to generate adequate pressure to function as an effective barrier."

Why do I have GERD?

GERD is a disease that is prevalent in economically developed areas of the world, particularly in North America, Europe, Japan, and Australia. Like over 190 million adults worldwide, you are probably wondering why you have GERD or acid reflux.

It is impossible to be certain as to why you have this disease and what is driving your symptoms. GERD occurs when the valve between the stomach and the esophagus is unable to generate adequate pressure to function as an effective barrier. Once the LES begins to deteriorate, stomach contents are able to reflux back up into the esophagus, resulting in the painful symptoms of GERD.

The LES can degrade or function abnormally due to a variety of causes such as overeating, hiatal hernia, pregnancy, and chemicals found in certain foods.

Our Diet is the Culprit

For many, the underlying reason for GERD is that we overeat! In many parts of the world, most people "eat to live." In economically developed countries, we "live to eat." In most economically developed countries the quality of food is so good that we crave more and more – and we eat more and more. In these areas, people are drawn to the typical American meal – double cheeseburgers and super-sized fries. Many adults, including many GERD sufferers, have become addicted to gaining satisfaction from a meal if and only if they feel full. Therein lies the problem.

What Happens When We Overeat?

When we eat more than a "comfortable" or appropriate amount of food for the stomach to handle, the stomach must stretch or distend to accommodate the additional volume. When this stretching happens, the lower end of the esophagus (where the LES is located) distends to form a shape that resembles the horn end of a trumpet. In this situation, the lower portions of the LES become exposed to stomach acid and resulting damage to the esophagus is possible. The stomach lining can accommodate acid that it normally produces for digestion. However, the esophagus and LES cannot handle contact with highly acidic stomach contents on a regular basis.

Overeating on a limited and intermittent basis is typically not a problem. These circumstances often result in minimal irritation of the lower esophagus and LES and the esophagus heals itself. However, repeated and significant overeating can damage the LES and cause it to lose its strength. Once the barrier is weakened, acid reflux occurs, initiating GERD symptoms.

How Distending the Stomach Impacts the Barrier Function of the LES

The LES has two properties that enable it to function as a barrier. These are the length of the LES and the pressure by which it "squeezes" the lower esophagus closed. If the LES is chronically exposed to acid as a result of stomach distension from overeating, it may become damaged to the point where it cannot generate pressure. As a result, BOTH the length of the LES is lost and its ability to generate pressure declines. As the barrier wears down, mild reflux symptoms may be intermittent. However, frequent reflux results in a significant reduction of both LES length and its ability to generate pressure over time. If ignored, it is possible that the LES's barrier function is not just reduced, but is essentially gone.

The obesity epidemic in the United States has created a very problematic situation. Obesity is generally the result of overeating; therefore, if you are obese the scenario described above is bound to occur. The increased pressure caused by large meals first compromises the function of the LES. Then, the very heavy abdominal wall compresses the stomach, resulting in excessive pressure on the LES. In fact, obese people are three times more likely to have frequent GERD than those that are not obese.

Your GERD symptoms are a message from your body telling you that something is wrong. Unless you take control of your illness and manage your disease, the messages may become more frequent and intense, and serious complications can result.

Lifestyle Choices Impact the LES

Certain lifestyle choices can also impact the effectiveness of the LES. Alcohol consumption is one such activity that has been studied and found to have a direct impact on the LES. Many heartburn sufferers report that their symptoms routinely occur after drinking alcohol. A study by Dr. Kaufman and Dr. Kay titled "Induction of gastro-esophageal reflux by alcohol," published in *GUT*, a peer-reviewed journal, found a strong correlation between alcohol consumption and GERD. In the study, healthy young adults were tested after consuming alcohol. Individuals were given either 180ml of vodka or 180ml of water to determine the impact of alcohol consumption on the LES. A significant difference was found between the two groups, and the researchers concluded that even small quantities of alcohol triggered GERD symptoms, even in healthy adults.

How significant is this issue? According to a Gallup survey conducted in July 2012, two thirds of all adults who responded to the survey reported that they consumed alcohol occasionally. Of these, twenty-two percent indicated that they "drank too much," representing an increase from seventeen percent the year before. Men reported more alcohol consumption, with an average of 6.2 drinks per week compared to women who reported consuming 2.2 drinks per week. Given the results of the study by Drs. Kaufman and Kay, it is clear that alcohol consumption may be a significant contributor to accelerating the growing incidence of GERD.

Smoking has also proven to be an important factor in reducing the LES's capabilities. Another article titled "Mechanisms of acid reflux associated with cigarette smoking," authored by Drs. Kahrilas and Gupta and published in *GUT*, studied smokers and nonsmokers. They concluded that, "cigarette smoking probably exacerbates reflux disease by directly provoking acid reflux and perhaps by a long-lasting reduction of the lower esophageal sphincter pressure." Although tobacco use in the U.S. has declined over the last twenty years, as reported by the CDC, nineteen percent of all U.S. adults still smoke cigarettes.

Given the current rates of obesity, alcohol consumption and tobacco use, it is surprising that only one in every three adults in the U.S. experiences GERD symptoms monthly. If we are unable to manage these trends in the future, it is clear that GERD will become an epidemic affecting more adults than any other chronic disease.

The Relationship Between Hiatal Hernias and GERD

A sliding hiatal hernia occurs when part of the stomach, which normally resides in the abdomen, moves upward through an enlarged opening in the diaphragm into the chest cavity. While there are other types of hiatal hernia, this is the type most commonly associated with GERD.

It is important to note that the presence of a hiatal hernia does not necessarily mean you have GERD. All patients with GERD do not have a hiatal hernia and all patients with a hiatal hernia do not have GERD! The term hiatal hernia simply describes a very common anatomic abnormality, one that often has no negative health consequences.

In some cases a hiatal hernia is the result of long-standing GERD, in which the hernia makes the preexisting "bad" LES worse (and GERD symptoms worsen as a result). In others, the hiatal hernia itself (rather than GERD, which may or may not be present) causes symptoms that mimic GERD. Finally, some people with a hiatal hernia have a normally functioning LES.

That being said, hiatal hernias can contribute to significant reflux due to the fact that the LES is no longer in its proper location in the abdomen. When the LES moves into the chest cavity, it no longer functions properly and remains open, allowing the acidic contents of the stomach to flow up into the esophagus. Unfortunately, this can be very painful. Symptoms associated with hiatal hernia include difficulty swallowing, a "full" feeling that sets in quickly during meals, and pain experienced immediately after eating. How a hiatal hernia is treated depends largely on which of the above situations exist.

Pregnancy and GERD

Reflux symptoms during pregnancy are a common complaint. In fact, about one half to two thirds of pregnant women experience GERD during pregnancy. This does not include those who are already being treated for this common condition with various OTC medications prior to becoming pregnant.

There are two main reasons that pregnant women experience the symptoms of reflux. Pregnancy changes the hormonal environment and the expanding uterus increases pressure in the abdomen. Both are thought to contribute to GERD. GERD and GERD-related symptoms resolve in most women after pregnancy, eliminating the need for treatment thereafter.

Recognize Your Role in Minimizing GERD

While certain potential causes of reflux (such as pregnancy and hiatal hernia) are not unhealthy, many reflux-inducing behaviors (such as overeating) should always be avoided. For example, eating supersized portions can have numerous adverse health effects and puts you at severe risk for GERD. Consuming large meals regularly increases your likelihood of becoming obese, which makes you **three times more likely to have GERD** than those who are not obese.

GERD is a long-term condition that varies in severity among sufferers. **GERD does not get better without making positive lifestyle changes.** If you are suffering from GERD, your goal should be to contain the disease and improve the quality of your life.

Chapter 4
The Symptoms That Say You Have GERD

"People with GERD experience a variety of symptoms in addition to the classic symptom of heartburn."

Classic Symptoms of GERD

GERD affects everyone differently. While it is only an occasional problem for some, GERD can be a lifestyle-limiting disease for many. It can disrupt daily activities, disturb sleep and decrease work productivity. People with GERD experience a variety of symptoms in addition to the classic symptom of heartburn. Unfortunately, symptoms can become more frequent and more severe over time, and can lead to serious complications if left unchecked. The most common symptoms of GERD are:

Heartburn

Heartburn is the classic GERD symptom. It is best described as a burning sensation in the chest and/or discomfort in the upper belly or abdomen, accompanied by a feeling of fullness. As the acidic stomach contents move up past the LES and gain contact with the esophagus, the resulting pain can range from mild to extremely severe. In some cases it can be confused with the symptoms of a heart attack.

Regurgitation

Regurgitation is hard to miss. It is the abrupt feeling of stomach contents rising past the esophagus and into the mouth. A horrible bitter taste and burning in the throat usually accompany this unpleasant surprise. This is often a significant warning sign of advanced reflux disease, indicating that your disease is severe.

Difficulty Swallowing (Dysphagia)

Although mild, difficulty swallowing is a symptom of GERD. More frequent or severe difficulty swallowing could be a symptom of esophageal cancer and should be promptly evaluated by an expert. Pressure and/or pain in the chest area, or the sensation that food is "stuck" in the throat are symptoms of dysphagia.

Chest Pain

GERD and heart disease share this symptom, and it can be very difficult to determine the real underlying cause of chest pain. Consequently, it is important to always seek immediate medical attention for chest pain to rule out a possible heart condition.

Symptoms You Probably Do Not Expect

There are several symptoms that most people do not realize may be related to GERD:

- Tooth decay, gingivitis and bad breath

- Earaches

- Asthma-like symptoms such as shortness of breath

- Recurring pneumonia

- Abdominal bloating and belching

Laryngopharyngeal Reflux (LPR)

For some people, the stomach contents can make their way all the way up the esophagus through the upper esophageal sphincter (UES) and into the throat and airway. This is known as laryngopharyngeal reflux, or LPR. LPR can cause symptoms such as chronic cough, throat clearing and hoarseness, either on their own or in conjunction with the more typical GERD symptoms.

Because these symptoms can be caused by so many other conditions, LPR is notoriously hard to diagnose. Unfortunately, there is no single test to confirm the diagnosis. The most widely used therapy for GERD is PPI medication; however, these powerful drugs are typically ineffective in the treatment of LPR. If you experience these symptoms, it is important that additional diagnostic tests be performed to confirm your GERD diagnosis.

Red Flags: Factors that Create Concern

"Alarm" symptoms, such as difficulty swallowing and/or chest pain, indicate the potential for serious complications and must be evaluated promptly. If you have experienced symptoms for more than five to ten years, you are at an increased risk for Barrett's esophagus, a precancerous condition. In these situations you must err on the side of caution and see a GERD expert to rule out any serious complications.

Chapter 5
The Stages of GERD: Why You Need To Know Yours

"Treatment options and recommendations for each stage are also different, so it is essential to know your stage before you begin any treatment plan."

GERD is a Chronic, Progressive Condition

GERD is a long-term chronic condition that varies in severity. Like many diseases, GERD has several stages ranging from mildly irritating to life threatening. Your goal should be to contain your disease while improving the quality of your life. The stages of GERD progression are best defined by symptoms in conjunction with tests, such as endoscopy, pH testing and biopsy.

Stage 1: Mild GERD

The majority of adults with GERD today have minor damage to their LES and experience mild GERD symptoms occasionally, roughly once or twice a month. In most cases they use OTC acid-suppressive medications such as antacids or H2 blockers at the onset of symptoms. Because their symptoms are controlled quickly, easily and inexpensively, their quality of life is unaffected. Here is an example:

> *"I am a forty-five-year-old man working as a traveling salesman for an auto parts company. Because of my job, I spend most of my time away from home and find myself eating fast food frequently. I have gained twenty-five pounds over the past twenty years but consider myself healthy. I started getting occasional episodes of discomfort under my breastbone about ten years ago. These lasted a short time and occurred almost every time I ate a double cheeseburger with fries and a large soda. I used to ignore these symptoms but the episodes have recently become more severe. They last longer and they are more frequent. I now have these problems about twice a week.*

> *Last week, I got up at night with a pain in my chest and I was worried that I was having a heart attack. The discomfort has increased since then and developed into a burning pain that I think is heartburn. I carry a packet of antacids in my pocket now and take a couple of these when the pain starts. Fortunately, the antacids control my symptoms very quickly and they are inexpensive. Now I take Tums before I eat a cheeseburger because I've found that this prevents the pain from recurring. My quality of life is pretty normal, except that I worry that I have a disease that may be serious. I have never experienced food regurgitation, I sleep at night lying flat in my bed, and I have never been to a physician."*

Stage 2: Moderate GERD

Stage 2 GERD is more difficult to control with acid-suppressive drugs and the accompanying reflux symptoms are more frequent and more intense. Damage to the LES is more extensive than that experienced in Stage 1. Many symptoms can be satisfactorily managed for the long term with more powerful acid-suppressive medications. Since many OTC antacids and H2 blockers often provide inadequate relief, prescription strength medications are necessary to manage the symptoms of acid reflux. Many can benefit from being treated by a knowledgeable GERD specialist. Here is an example:

> *"I am a forty-three-year-old woman working as an executive in a commercial bank, managing real estate loans. My weight is in proportion to my height and I exercise several times each week to maintain my weight level. I started getting heartburn during my second pregnancy, seven years ago. Although the symptoms decreased after my baby was born, they did not completely disappear. In fact, over the last three years they have increased significantly. I now get an episode almost every day, which is troubling to me. I am afraid to eat normally and have changed my eating habits. I also wake up frequently at night with a pain in my chest that goes away quickly when I sit up.*
>
> *I have tried a variety of acid-suppressive drugs that I purchased at the pharmacy, but even the recommended dosage of Prilosec OTC did not fully control my symptoms. I went to my family doctor who prescribed a stronger drug that I use daily and my symptoms have improved, but they are not resolved. I am still afraid of eating and I sleep with two pillows to avoid the burning sensation I sometimes get at night. I would say that my life is generally alright but not perfect. I still have occasional episodes of regurgitation but I don't consider them to be too troublesome. My family doctor has told me that there is nothing more that can be done for me. Surgery is the only alternative to drug treatment and my family doctor had little to offer concerning that alternative. I have not seen a GERD specialist and have never had an endoscopic exam or any other testing for my problem."*

Stage 3: Severe GERD

Stage 3 GERD results in a substantially lower quality of life and is considered a very serious problem. Even prescription acid-suppressive drugs do not control symptoms to the individual's satisfaction and regurgitation is frequent. It is also likely that one or more of the complications associated with erosive GERD may be present. It is highly recommended that anyone with severe GERD schedule a thorough examination by a knowledgeable GERD specialist. Here is an example:

"I am a fifty-two-year-old man and I work in a car dealership as a salesman. I am moderately overweight but certainly not obese. I have had heartburn on and off for the past twenty years. Until I was put on a prescription medication by my gastroenterologist, I experienced heartburn almost daily. I have been to numerous physicians that have performed a variety of tests, including endoscopic evaluation of my throat. Although my daily prescription acid-suppressive drugs worked well for many years, over the last two years I have developed frequent regurgitation. I can no longer sleep in my bed and for the last nine months I've been forced to sleep in my recliner. I am afraid to eat, knowing that I will develop heartburn followed by regurgitation. Last week I awoke in the middle of the night with an episode of coughing and shortness of breath. This really scared me because I thought I was suffocating. I spoke with my gastroenterologist the next day. He told me not to worry and recommended continuation of my prescription drugs. When I asked him about surgical options, he told me that he would prefer for me to continue with my current treatment plan."

Stage 4: Pre-Cancerous Condition or Reflux-Induced Esophageal Cancer

Stage 4 is the result of many years of severe reflux. Ten to fifteen percent of long-term sufferers progress to this very advanced condition. Due to long-term reflux, the lining of the esophagus has been damaged, resulting in cellular changes. It should be noted that these cellular changes could develop in some people with only minimal symptoms. Stage 4 involves the development of a precancerous condition called Barrett's esophagus or a more severe condition called dysplasia. These conditions are not cancers, but raise the risk of developing reflux-induced esophageal cancer. **Many people with Stage 4 GERD have no pain or warning signs!** At this stage, typical GERD symptoms may also be accompanied by burning in the throat, chronic cough and hoarseness. Stricture, or a narrowing of the esophagus, can also occur. This is characterized by the sensation that food is sticking in the esophagus. This symptom can also be caused by esophageal cancer. Stage 4 GERD can only be diagnosed with an endoscopic examination and a biopsy of cells taken from the lower esophagus. RefluxMD highly recommends that Stage 4 disease be cared for in an ongoing way by a knowledgeable GERD specialist. Here is an example:

"I am a sixty-two-year-old male who retired two years ago. I have had heartburn for fifteen years and my symptoms were controlled with acid-suppressive drugs, until last year when I began to experience regurgitation that is getting worse monthly. I also developed a troublesome and constant cough and my voice has become hoarse.

Last month, my physician referred me to a gastroenterologist who performed an endoscopic examination on my throat and I was told that I had Barrett's esophagus. He told me that, while Barrett's esophagus indicated an increased risk of cancer, the risk was very small and that I should not worry. He increased my dosage of acid-suppressive drugs and told me that I needed annual endoscopic examinations. I asked him if I had any other options and he mentioned surgery. However, he indicated that he would prefer to monitor me and he would suggest that alternative only if necessary."

Each of these stages is unique; however, transition from stage to stage is not clearly defined and noticeable. Treatment options and recommendations for each stage are also different, so it is essential to know your stage before you begin any treatment plan.

Chapter 6
Complications if GERD is not Treated Properly

"The risk of developing esophageal cancer is small, but also very real."

GERD: More than a nuisance

Do you consider GERD to be "just a nuisance"? This is one of the most common myths that we hear about this chronic condition. While it may be just an annoyance for some, for others it can have a dramatic impact on quality of life and can lead to more serious complications. Symptoms can be so severe that sufferers are unable to sleep horizontally in a bed and can only sleep upright in a chair. In other cases individuals are unable to eat normal meals, since they tend to immediately regurgitate their food. In its most advanced stages, chronic acid reflux can result in esophagitis, throat ulcers, strictures (narrowing of the esophagus), Barrett's esophagus (a precancerous condition), and reflux-induced adenocarcinoma (esophageal cancer).

At the outset, several facts should be emphasized:

1. Deaths from esophageal cancer are on the rise, yet this diagnosis comprises a small percentage of all adults with GERD symptoms. However, the probability of being diagnosed with cancer increases with each of the following risk factors: males, age of fifty-five or older, disease term of over ten years, smoking, drinking, obesity, and/or a diagnosis of Barrett's esophagus.

2. The very small risk of getting cancer has made physicians complacent. The management guidelines for treating GERD basically ignore the risk of cancer. While this may be appropriate, it is a devastating policy for the approximately 20,000 people who are destined to get esophageal cancer in 2015. No effort is made by present treatment guidelines to identify those at risk and to assist them to do whatever possible to decrease their chances of premature death. This policy is certainly not optimal, and researchers are working to identify indicators that predict those who are more likely to get cancer.

3. There is evidence of an effective method to decrease the likelihood of death from GERD-induced cancer. This involves detecting a premalignant condition called Barrett's esophagus by performing endoscopy and biopsy tests. Once Barrett's esophagus is identified, putting those individuals on medical surveillance facilitates early detection of cancer if it occurs. Early detection allows treatment by minimally invasive techniques rather than major surgery. As with many cancers, early detection increases the chance of a cure.

Long-term Symptoms Increase the Likelihood of Complications

Unfortunately, endoscopy cannot be recommended for everyone displaying symptoms of GERD, due to the excessive cost burden on the U.S. healthcare system. However, we can identify high risk factors that increase the likelihood of progressing to Barrett's esophagus. One such risk factor is the duration of this disease. Those experiencing symptoms for more than ten years should view this as a significant warning flag, regardless of the strength of the symptoms. It should be noted that stronger and more frequent symptoms present a greater likelihood of progressing to Barrett's esophagus and/or cancer in the future.

Complications from Chronic Acid Reflux
Esophagitis

The esophagus is the tube of muscles that contracts and moves food from the throat to the stomach. When stomach acid repeatedly comes into contact with the lining of the esophagus it can damage that sensitive tissue, causing esophageal redness, tenderness and swelling. This inflammation is called esophagitis. If reflux continues untreated, esophagitis may progress to bleeding of the esophagus, ulcers and scarring. This type of damage is reversible and can be treated by reducing the acidity of the stomach contents with acid-reducing medications.

Esophageal Erosions (Ulcers)

Esophageal erosions indicate the slow but sure breakdown of the esophagus. Stomach acid can wear away tissues in the esophagus, causing an open wound. This wound is known as an erosion or ulcer and may bleed, cause pain and make it hard to swallow. As with esophagitis, acid-reducing medications can help the esophagus to heal.

Strictures

Exposure to acid from refluxed stomach contents can cause damage to cells in the lower esophagus, which may cause scar tissue to form. When the damaged lining of the esophagus becomes scarred it sometimes causes the esophagus to narrow. This is called a stricture. These strictures get in the way of eating and drinking by stopping food and drink from traveling to the stomach. Strictures can be treated with dilation, using an instrument to carefully stretch and expand the opening in the esophagus.

Barrett's Esophagus

One serious complication of GERD is Barrett's esophagus, in which the tissue covering the esophagus morphs into tissue that looks like the tissue lining the stomach and intestines. Some people with Barrett's esophagus have GERD symptoms while others do not have any symptoms at all. Barrett's esophagus is a precancerous condition that leads to increased risk of developing esophageal adenocarcinoma. People who have Barrett's esophagus are between 30 to 125 times more predisposed to develop esophageal cancer than those who do not.

If you have had reflux symptoms or have taken antireflux medications for over ten years, regardless of any other factors, consider undergoing endoscopy testing to determine if you have Barrett's esophagus. This is an important screening test for those at risk. In most cases the results of this test will be negative, but this is valuable information nonetheless. If you have Barrett's esophagus, then you should establish a "surveillance protocol," which will improve your chances of survival if you are one of the unlucky people who develops esophageal cancer. The most common form of surveillance is observation with repeated endoscopies as often as once every one to three years. The objective is to detect the progression of any abnormality that could indicate a transition to cancer. Early identification of dysplasia (low-grade and high-grade) or even an early stage cancer offers an enhanced chance of treating the abnormality, versus later-stage detection.

Ablation for Barrett's Esophagus

Other management strategies for Barrett's esophagus have been developed besides the traditional surveillance program. The most recent and promising is radiofrequency ablation (RFA), also referred to as ablation or HALO. This procedure involves using highly controlled radiofrequency energy to eliminate or "ablate" the areas where Barrett's has developed in the normal lining of the esophagus. Once the Barrett's tissue is eliminated, the normal lining of the esophagus regenerates over several months.

Is Ablation Effective?

Extensive research suggests that RFA can either prevent or delay the progression of Barrett's esophagus to a more serious state, including cancer. However, follow-up endoscopies at specific time intervals are recommended, usually six months, two years, or three years following the procedure. Since this procedure has been used by medical professionals for less than twenty years, sufficient evidence has not been gathered to conclusively prove that RFA prevents cancer. To date, the medical literature supports the premise that RFA makes the development of cancer less likely. The caveat is that ablation must be performed by an experienced physician on patients who will reliably return for follow-up endoscopies and be retreated if necessary.

If you are diagnosed with Barrett's esophagus, it is important that you understand the condition, the associated risk of cancer, and the management options available to you.

Esophageal Cancer (Esophageal Adenocarcinoma)

Esophageal adenocarcinoma is a cancer of the esophagus that can be caused by GERD.

While esophageal adenocarcinoma is rare, the incidence of this deadly disease has increased sixfold in the last forty years. What's worse is that esophageal adenocarcinoma is one of the most lethal types of cancer in humans. Approximately eighty-five percent of those who develop esophageal cancer die of their disease, often within one to two years of diagnosis. Early detection is the key to effectively treating this cancer. Those with esophageal cancer might not be aware of any signs or symptoms at first. In more advanced stages, symptoms of esophageal cancer include difficulty swallowing, weight loss, pain behind the breastbone, coughing, hoarseness, indigestion and heartburn.

Avoiding Complications from Chronic Acid Reflux

The best way to prevent the complications that may come from chronic acid reflux is to get your condition under control. The odds of damage to the esophagus from acid reflux are reduced when there are fewer acid reflux episodes. While acid-reducing medications can minimize symptoms and help to heal esophagitis and erosions, they do not stop reflux from happening. This may mean that you also need to make some changes to your lifestyle. Many people can reduce the incidence of symptoms considerably by knowing and avoiding heartburn triggers and avoiding behaviors that play a part in acid reflux.

If you have experienced symptoms for over ten years, particular diligence and awareness of your disease is recommended. It is now time for you to take ownership and control of your disease and determine if you have Barrett's esophagus. This is true whether or not your symptoms are controlled by drug therapy. Medications do not stop the progression of GERD and do not significantly decrease your risk of developing Barrett's esophagus or adenocarcinoma.

It's also important that you be alert to changes in your health. Signs that your GERD could be getting worse include regurgitation of food, difficulty swallowing, sore throat and hoarseness. If you notice any of these symptoms, be sure to let your doctor know. Do not wait until it is too late. Take control of your chronic acid reflux today, so you feel better now AND down the road.

Chapter 7
The Importance of Accurate Diagnostic Testing

"GERD cannot be diagnosed based upon symptoms; accurate diagnostic tests are essential to confirm or rule out reflux disease."

Why Testing Matters

Seventy percent of adults with reflux disease have never seen a physician. They self-diagnose and often self-medicate. Of those who *have* seen a physician, approximately seventy percent have only seen a primary care physician who is not an expert on GERD and does not have the diagnostic tools to confirm an accurate diagnosis. GERD cannot be diagnosed based upon symptoms; accurate diagnostic tests are essential to confirm or rule out reflux disease.

When you see a physician who is an expert on GERD about your reflux symptoms, a variety of tests may be used to evaluate your condition. In combination, these procedures provide a complete evaluation; each has a purpose and each represents a different piece of the puzzle. These procedures only provide complete clarity if they are coordinated and conducted properly. All too often, an incomplete evaluation results in a patient gaining no further insight into their condition.

Common Diagnostic Tests

The following are the most commonly used tests when evaluating a patient with GERD-like symptoms:

Upper Endoscopy

An upper endoscopy or esophagogastroduodenoscopy (EGD) provides a visual examination of the esophagus and stomach. An endoscope is a thin, flexible tube with a tiny, light, video camera on the end. During the procedure, the patient is sedated while the doctor advances the endoscope into the esophagus and stomach, and inspects the tissue via images on a video monitor. This diagnostic test allows doctors to see any areas of inflammation or irritation and rule out many other conditions. It is important to note that EGD alone cannot definitively diagnose GERD.

Biopsies

During an upper endoscopy a doctor may perform a biopsy to take small tissue samples from areas that appear abnormal. A pathologist will examine these tissue samples under a microscope to determine if the cells show any signs of change, also referred to as dysplasia.

Ambulatory pH Testing

Considered the gold standard of testing for GERD, ambulatory pH testing is the most accurate and objective test for diagnosing GERD, because it actually measures acid levels in the esophagus. During the test, a small sensor is placed in the esophagus. Once in place, the sensor measures pH levels over a twenty-four to forty-eight-hour period. Once completed, the test shows the effect that meals, daily activities and sleep have on the pH levels in the esophagus that contribute to acid reflux.

Esophageal Manometry

Esophageal manometry is a test used to gauge the ability of the esophagus and LES to effectively move food towards the stomach. This test measures the pressure in the esophagus as a patient swallows, allowing doctors to detect any abnormalities in the underlying anatomy of the esophagus. Manometry can detect a hiatal hernia and damage to the LES, as well as other conditions that may mimic GERD. Manometry or alternative testing to assess the motility of the esophagus is required if surgery is being considered as a treatment option.

Barium Swallow

A barium swallow involves an x-ray examination of the esophagus, stomach and upper part of the small intestines. Sometimes called an upper GI series, this procedure requires that the patient drink a contrast medium called barium, which coats the intestinal tract and makes it possible to see the anatomy on x-rays. A barium swallow helps the medical team to identify hiatal hernias, tumors or areas of inflammation of the esophagus and stomach.

What You Should do if Your GERD Symptoms Persist

Too often, treatment for GERD begins and ends with a prescription for PPIs. If you continue to have symptoms even while on medication or if you are concerned about taking medications long-term, it is time to pursue more aggressive testing to gain a complete understanding of your condition. Studies have shown that thirty-two percent of all PPI users are not refluxing and should not be using these powerful medications. In most cases, these individuals were either self-diagnosed or diagnosed by a physician based upon a discussion of symptoms alone. Unless definitive diagnostic tests are performed, you cannot be confident that you have GERD and you are unable to make appropriate treatment decisions.

Chapter 8
Lifestyle Choices to Treat GERD

"Lifestyle choices are recommended for anyone with reflux disease regardless of stage, since they have been proven to provide some level of symptom relief."

Lifestyle Choices can Relieve Symptoms

In general, there are three categories of treatment for GERD: medication, procedural interventions and lifestyle choices. Lifestyle choices are recommended for anyone with reflux disease regardless of stage, since they have been proven to provide some level of symptom relief. However, as GERD progresses, these activities alone may not provide adequate relief. Therefore, if you think you may have GERD, it is important to start these lifestyle changes as early as possible.

Manage Your Weight: Target a Healthy BMI

Weight gain increases the risk of GERD. Consuming too much food often causes individuals to become obese. It also causes the stomach to distend frequently, damaging the LES and leading to reflux. To make things worse, obese people carry excess weight in the abdominal wall, which increases pressure on the abdomen and LES. Adjusting dietary intake with the goal of reducing weight will most likely reduce your heartburn. For some, even the loss of five or ten pounds may make a substantial difference. For those who are very overweight (with a BMI greater than 35), weight loss surgery may be an option to consider. Some of these procedures, such as gastric bypass surgery, can help to control reflux and reduce GERD symptoms in addition to assisting in weight loss.

Limit the Size of Your Meal Portions

Portion control is on the top of every GERD expert's list. Overeating is an activity that can put excess pressure on the LES. One way to manage your portions is to eat small meals more frequently and to stop eating when you feel full.

Avoid Your Trigger Foods

There are many common foods that may trigger heartburn and other GERD symptoms, but everyone is different. You should identify those foods and beverages that drive *your* symptoms. Once you recognize that certain foods or beverages create symptoms (such as coffee, chocolate, citrus, etc.), avoid those foods and plan your meals accordingly.

Eat Dinner Earlier

Since it takes several hours for a meal to digest in your stomach, eating earlier in the evening allows that meal to break down and move out of the stomach before you recline for sleep. Avoid late night snacks, since they can restart the digestive process for a few hours.

If You Smoke, Stop Immediately

Smoking contributes to the weakening of the LES that encourages reflux. Smoking has been proven to be a risk factor for multiple cancers, including esophageal cancer and lung cancer. Quitting smoking is not easy. In section five, we address specific strategies designed to help you overcome the smoking obstacle.

Reduce or Eliminate Alcohol Consumption

Research has proven that alcohol reduces the barrier function of the LES and can cause GERD symptoms. This research has also confirmed that consuming large volumes of alcohol has an increased impact on GERD symptoms.

Give up or Limit Carbonated Beverages

Carbonation is another factor that can distend the stomach and put pressure on the LES. If you cannot give up carbonated drinks completely, avoid drinking them during meals and in the evening.

Avoid Tight-fitting Clothes

Tight clothes, waistbands or belts put pressure on the abdomen that can mimic the same LES pressure that exists with obese or overweight individuals as noted above.

Diaphragm Exercises

As stated earlier, the LES is the barrier between the stomach and the esophagus that prevents reflux. The LES is augmented and surrounded by the diaphragm. Unlike the LES, an involuntary muscle that cannot be strengthened by exercise, the diaphragm is a voluntary muscle that can be made stronger by exercise. Although clinical research has yet to prove that exercising the diaphragm will improve the LES's barrier capabilities, the following exercise is not potentially harmful and may provide a reduction of symptoms.

Diaphragm exercise is a conscious breathing technique that uses the diaphragm rather than the lungs and the chest to create each breath. It entails expanding the abdomen to inhale and then contracting the abdomen without exhaling. Do this abdominal exercise five to ten times and then exhale. Repeat this process ten times in a row. It may help to place your hands on your abdomen to maintain focus on the expansion and contraction of your stomach. This exercise can be done sitting, standing or lying down. Proceed with caution at least initially, since deep, excessive breathing can induce hyperventilation. If you feel lightheaded at any time, stop the exercise and wait to attempt it again until the next day.

Sleep and GERD Symptoms

If GERD is impacting your sleep, here are several recommendations that you should consider:

- Try sleeping on your <u>left side</u> rather than the right side of your body, or on your back or stomach.

- Raise the head of your bed by placing books or a brick under the headboard. The upper part of the bed only needs to be elevated five to seven inches for this to be effective.

- Extra pillows or commercially available foam wedges tend to work poorly, since they bend the neck rather than elevating the entire chest.

- Stay in an upright position, either sitting or standing, for at least ninety minutes after dinner.

- Do not go to bed for at least three hours after a meal. Although this may be a difficult recommendation to follow, it has proven to be very effective in reducing heartburn symptoms.

A Note About LPR and Lifestyle

LPR, or laryngopharyngeal reflux, is often treated with acid-reducing medications like PPIs. Unfortunately, LPR symptoms do not always respond as well to medications as traditional GERD symptoms. As a result, diet and lifestyle modifications to minimize reflux like those suggested above are a key part of your treatment if you struggle with those symptoms. In addition, people with LPR should avoid drying the throat. Drink plenty of water and avoid foods, beverages and medications that can cause dehydration like caffeine, alcohol and antihistamines.

While diet and lifestyle modifications can certainly help, they are only as good as your ability to stick with them. We were excited to learn about a new device designed specifically to help people struggling to control their LPR symptoms – the Reza Band®. The Reza Band®, approved by the FDA in March 2015, is a wearable acid reflux control device designed to stop the flow of stomach contents through the upper esophageal sphincter (UES). Worn while you sleep, the Reza Band® increases pressure in the UES to stop reflux while you wear it. Studies have shown that it can significantly reduce the symptoms of LPR within the first two weeks of use. Though the device is new and more long-term data is needed to assess its efficacy, it seems the Reza Band® could be a promising first line of defense for people with LPR.

Chapter 9
Using Medications to Treat GERD

"When considering medication as a treatment option for reflux disease, remember that no drug can provide permanent relief."

Make an Informed Decision

The use of prescription and OTC medications in the U.S. is at an all-time high. According to a Mayo Clinic study[1], nearly seventy percent of Americans take at least one prescription drug daily and more than half take two or more. It is safe to say that American society is overmedicated today. Many medications help people to live longer and happier lives – insulin for diabetics and antibiotics for infections are excellent examples. However, the use of medications for the treatment of many chronic conditions may not be appropriate, and in many cases patients are unaware of the potentially harmful effects of these pharmaceutical drugs. For some, diet, exercise and lifestyle modifications are more effective for prevention (and often treatment) of the underlying conditions and/or the diseases themselves than use of pharmaceuticals. If you are considering using daily maintenance medications, it is essential to know as much as possible about the risks and benefits of these drugs in order to make an informed decision with your physician.

About Antireflux Medications

A brief search online may lead you to believe permanent relief from GERD is just a quick pill or chewable tablet away. While numerous medications are available for relieving the symptoms of reflux disease, be aware that these drugs are incapable of directly treating its root cause – a defective LES. Unable to actually prevent the backflow of stomach contents into your LES, these medications function instead by neutralizing or reducing the amount of acid produced by the stomach. Because this treatment approach aims to control symptoms rather than addressing the cause of the disease, the long-term management of reflux disease through use of medications alone often fails. However, it is important to note that medications may play an important role in improving patient wellness when used correctly.

Types of Reflux Medications
Acid Neutralizers

Examples: Tums, Rolaids, Maalox, Mylanta, Alka-Seltzer

Acid neutralizers represent one of the most common types of drugs used to treat

---

[1] *Mayo News Releases. "Nearly 7 in 10 Americans Take Prescription Drugs, Mayo Clinic, Olmsted Medical Find." 19 June 2013*

reflux disease. These OTC medications are basic compounds (i.e. alkaline or high pH) like calcium carbonate that provide temporary relief from symptoms by neutralizing stomach acid. They are used during reflux episodes or before eating a meal that is likely to cause heartburn. They reduce the acid level in the stomach immediately (albeit for a short period of time), and if used in sufficient dosages, can reduce the stomach acid pH level enough to reduce GERD symptoms when reflux occurs.

Your stomach is constantly monitoring and adjusting its pH level for optimal digestion. Therefore, it responds to the change in pH level caused by acid neutralizers by quickly ramping up acid secretion, in order to bring the pH back to the body's normal level. As a result, acid neutralizers only relieve symptoms for a short period of time. The fact that these drugs have had a large percentage of the market for over five decades suggests that they are effective in controlling reflux symptoms with intermittent use.

Benefits of Acid Reducers

- Readily available over the counter
- Inexpensive
- Provide quick relief of mild symptoms
- Can relieve symptoms during a reflux episode
- Can prevent heartburn if taken before a meal that is known to produce heartburn
- Safe

Concerns About Acid Reducers

- Short duration of symptom relief
- Ineffective in long-term management of symptoms
- Ineffective in relieving moderate to severe symptoms

Side Effects of Acid Reducers

Few side effects have been associated with acid neutralizers. In fact, some that contain calcium in their formula can actually act as nutritional calcium supplements.

Histamine-2 Receptor Antagonists (H2 Blockers)

Examples: Pepcid, Zantac, Tagamet, cimetidine, ranitidine

H2 blockers are a category of drugs that work by deactivating the cellular receptors within the stomach responsible for signaling the production of acid. When H-2 receptors are blocked, acid secretion by the cells in the stomach is decreased. If reflux occurs while this blockage is in place, the likelihood of heartburn is decreased. These drugs take longer to reduce gastric acid than acid neutralizers, but they produce a more sustained acid reduction. H2 blockers are less effective than PPIs in suppressing acid secretion on a long-term basis, but they act more quickly to reduce acid than PPIs. They are sometimes used in conjunction with PPIs to augment the efficacy of those drugs.

Benefits of H2 Blockers

- Readily available over the counter
- Provide longer-term relief from symptoms than acid neutralizers
- Act more quickly than PPIs in reducing acid secretion
- Less expensive than PPIs
- Fewer complications than PPIs

Concerns About H2 Blockers

- Less effective than PPIs in the long term
- Ineffective in relieving severe symptoms because the total amount of acid reduction achieved is much lower than that of PPIs

Side Effects of H2 Blockers

Few side effects have been associated with Histamine-2 receptor antagonists, with the exception of cimetidine. Users of this variant of the medication have been known to experience hypotension, headaches, fatigue, dizziness, confusion, constipation, diarrhea, and/or rash.

Proton Pump Inhibitors (PPIs)

Examples: Prilosec, Prevacid, Zegarid, Nexium, Protonix, omeprazole, esomeprazole, lansoprazole

PPIs provide the most powerful method for decreasing acid production in the stomach. PPIs work by inhibiting the proton pumps in the stomach's acid-producing cells. When used correctly, PPIs can provide relief from acid reflux for fourteen to eighteen hours each day. PPIs typically require three to four days to begin working and are not very useful when taken to control symptoms as they occur. These drugs are generally prescribed for a period of two weeks or longer. To be effective, PPIs need to be used continuously to keep acid levels low, so that the damage and symptoms are lessened when acid reflux inevitably occurs.

Benefits of PPIs

- Most powerful option for relief of acid reflux symptoms because they achieve the best control of acid secretion available

- Provide longer-term relief from symptoms than other medications

Concerns About PPIs

- FDA warning labels describe concerns with long-term use of PPIs that include an increased risk of bone fractures, vitamin B12 deficiency, magnesium deficiency and increased incidence of *Clostridium difficile* infections

- May increase severity of symptoms if treatment is discontinued because of rebound acid secretion

- Ineffective for quickly treating symptoms as they occur

- Do not address the cause of reflux disease – LES damage is permanent and not reversed by PPIs

- Do not prevent Barrett's esophagus or cancer

Side Effects of PPIs

Direct side effects may include headaches, diarrhea and abdominal pain. Long-term side effects may include interactions with other medications and increased risk of hip fracture or *Clostridium difficile* infection.

No Drug can Provide Permanent Relief

When considering medication as a treatment option for reflux disease, remember that no drug can provide permanent relief. Though these medications can help to control symptoms, they do not address the cause of acid reflux: a damaged or defective LES. Additionally, complications of reflux disease such as Barrett's esophagus and esophageal cancer are not addressed through the use of medication. Remember, improving your diet, losing weight and making other lifestyle modifications can have a profound effect on your day-to-day symptoms and overall health without exposing you to potential side effects or health complications. Consult your doctor before beginning and/or stopping any drug treatment regimen for reflux disease.

Chapter 10
Surgical Alternatives for GERD

"The objective of the surgical and endoscopic procedures for GERD is to restore the integrity of the damaged LES to stop reflux."

Surgical Alternatives to Repair the LES

Unlike acid-suppressive medical therapy, the objective of the surgical and endoscopic procedures for GERD is to restore the integrity of the damaged LES to stop reflux. This consists of augmenting or repairing the LES's function to restore its barrier capabilities and achieve a permanent correction. Surgical alternatives should reduce or eliminate symptoms and stop stomach contents from reaching the esophagus. The goal is to stop all reflux, which can be validated by a postoperative pH study. The complete cessation of reflux will result in the elimination of GERD symptoms and the elimination of the need for medications. However, even if reflux is not completely eliminated, the occurrence of symptoms and use of medications should be significantly reduced. With each procedure, the desired outcome must be balanced with risks, side effects and durability.

Laparoscopic Procedures
Nissen Fundoplication

The "gold standard" to which all antireflux procedures are compared is laparoscopic Nissen fundoplication. This minimally-invasive surgical procedure is performed under general anesthesia via several small incisions. A slender scope (called a laparoscope) is inserted into the abdomen. It produces a high-resolution image on a monitor that the surgeon observes as he performs the procedure. The procedure involves repairing the hiatal hernia that is typically present, and recreating a functional valve by wrapping part of the stomach around the lower esophagus at the site of the LES. The procedure takes approximately one to two hours with an overnight stay in the hospital afterwards. Most people are back to light everyday activity within a week. A successful laparoscopic Nissen fundoplication stops the reflux approximately eighty to eighty-five percent of the time and ninety percent of all patients typically remain satisfied with the procedure after five years. Side effects may include excess gas and bloating, as well as the permanent inability to belch or vomit. The Nissen procedure stops reflux more reliably than any other existing therapies.

LINX Reflux Management System

The FDA approved the LINX Reflux Management System in March 2012. This procedure is performed using the same minimally-invasive technique as the Nissen; however, it is much less complex and may be performed on an outpatient basis that does not require an overnight stay at the hospital. The LINX device is a specially designed "bracelet" of magnetic beads that is placed loosely around the esophagus, augmenting the damaged LES. As food is swallowed, it passes into the stomach and the magnetic beads separate, allowing the food to pass into the stomach and then close again, thus preventing reflux. The procedure takes approximately thirty minutes. The results are similar to that of the Nissen procedure, but with minimal side effects. Presently, this procedure is only available at select medical centers but availability is expected to expand quickly. This procedure is also reversible. Since the LINX procedure is new, long-term outcome data is unavailable.

Endoscopic Procedures

There are several procedures designed to repair the LES. They are performed orally (through the mouth) and are classified as endoscopic antireflux procedures. There are no abdominal incisions. Several of these types of procedures have been introduced in recent years and RefluxMD will comment on them as clinical evidence becomes available.

Transoral Intraluminal Fundoplication

Transoral intraluminal fundoplication (TIF), sometimes referred to as Esophyx, is one such procedure that is available today. Under general anesthesia, a special endoscope is used to perform a partial fundoplication from inside the stomach. This procedure has been available for several years and improves GERD symptoms in most patients. It is not as effective as the Nissen fundoplication, but it improves symptoms and decreases the need for medication in most patients with few side effects. Additionally, the potential side effects of the TIF procedure are substantially less than that of the Nissen, making it attractive to many who are seeking a surgical solution. A similar procedure called the MUSE system by Medigus was approved by the FDA in 2014.

Stretta

The Stretta procedure uses radiofrequency waves to remodel tissue and improve muscle tone in the LES. This procedure involves lowering a radiofrequency transmitter device through the esophagus to the LES. Once in place, a mini balloon inflates and begins to deliver radiofrequency energy to the muscle tissue. The patient is under conscious sedation while the procedure is being administered and is able to return to their normal lifestyle the following day, without any overnight stays in the hospital. The full impact of the Stretta technique is not realized until two to six months after the procedure, when the esophagus is fully healed.

Research your options

Understanding each of the available surgical and endoscopic treatments for GERD is difficult. Conflicting information and data exists about each procedure and the information you receive may be confusing at times. You should contact a reflux expert for further education on these procedures. A qualified GERD surgeon will discuss the facts regarding each treatment alternative so that you can make an informed decision. If you elect a surgical alternative, the procedure should be performed by a GERD expert with a documented high-level of success.

Chapter 11
Home Remedies to Manage Your Symptoms

"Some patients claim they are able to manage their symptoms through treatments not found in the neighborhood pharmacy. Instead, many pay a visit to their home pantries."

Alternatives to Western Medicine

When choosing a treatment for acid reflux, alternatives to traditional pharmaceuticals are often overlooked or ignored. While medications are the most common treatment method for reflux, some patients claim they are able to manage their symptoms through treatments not found in the neighborhood pharmacy. Instead, many pay a visit to their home pantries.

The following list provides an overview of several home remedies that have been reported to reduce the symptoms of reflux. Since everyone is different, it is not possible to predict if these will work for you. Scientific research into the effectiveness of these alternative treatments is ongoing and the evidence to date is largely anecdotal – with the exception of baking soda and chewing gum. Though some individuals have reported relief from heartburn with alternative remedies, consult your doctor before trying any of these. There is always the possibility that your symptoms could be caused by something other than GERD and using these remedies could delay finding the definitive cause.

Baking Soda

Similar to many acid reflux medications, baking soda alleviates symptoms by reducing the acidity of stomach acid. A proven alternative treatment, the alkalinity of baking soda allows it to temporarily neutralize stomach acid, resulting in less painful and noticeable symptoms if the stomach contents reflux into the esophagus. To try this remedy, dissolve a heaping teaspoon of baking soda in eight to twelve ounces of water and drink the mixture. There are some drawbacks – First, this remedy tastes terrible! Try adding a touch of honey or sugar to offset the unpleasant taste of the baking soda. Second, the overuse of baking soda can produce an excess of digestive gases, resulting in increased belching, bloating, stomach cramps and slight pain or discomfort.

Gum Chewing

Temporary relief from reflux symptoms might be as simple as following up a meal with a stick of gum. Independent scientific studies have found that patients who chewed gum for thirty to sixty minutes immediately after meals experienced a noticeable decrease in symptoms. It is believed that the increased production of saliva caused by chewing gum has the effect of clearing acidic and potentially painful reflux contents from the esophagus. Additionally, the alkaline nature of saliva can help to neutralize the stomach acid before it passes into the esophagus. It is also recommended to avoid peppermint or spearmint-flavored chewing gum, since they are known to make symptoms worse.

Apple Cider Vinegar

As someone who experiences the unpleasant and often painful symptoms of acid reflux, the idea of consuming an acidic substance like apple cider vinegar might not sound appealing. Yet, many individuals swear by its effectiveness in alleviating symptoms. Despite anecdotal evidence of apple cider vinegar's effectiveness, the science behind these claims has not been substantiated due to a lack of research on the subject. Some believe that by helping to balance the stomach's acidity, the vinegar may prevent the stomach from overcompensating by creating excess acid. Be warned – the taste of this remedy makes it difficult to drink. Mixing a tablespoon of apple cider vinegar with honey and water can make this home remedy easier to swallow.

Ginger

Used as an herbal treatment for a variety of ailments, ginger is sometimes taken to alleviate acid reflux symptoms. While there is no hard scientific evidence to suggest that ginger has any effect on reflux, it is thought to have a calming effect on digestion, thus giving some users relief. A warm cup of ginger tea is a simple and relaxing way to consume this natural medicine. Just be sure to avoid ginger teas containing caffeine as it can make your symptoms worse.

Probiotic Supplements

If you have visited the dairy section of your local grocery store lately, it is likely that you have come across probiotics. Typically found in yogurts and fermented foods, probiotics are living organisms that are thought to be beneficial to the body's digestive system. Research into the potential benefits of probiotics for reflux is ongoing. However, some researchers[2] have theorized that a daily probiotic supplement can strengthen the lining of the gastrointestinal (GI) tract, potentially protecting it from harmful bacteria and excess acid.

Chili Peppers

Chili peppers have been used as a digestive aid in cultures around the world for centuries. Capsaicin, the compound in peppers responsible for their heat, has been shown to relieve pain and itching, and fight inflammation. One study[3] even found that capsaicin seems to slow the growth of prostate cancer. So what does this have to do

---

[2] *National for Complementary and Integrative Health. "Oral Probiotics: An Introduction." January 2007. Last Updated December 2012.*

[3] *Díaz-Laviada I. 1Department of Biochemistry & Molecular Biology, School of Medicine, University of Alcala, Alcalá de Henares, 28871 Madrid, Spain. "Effect of capsaicin on prostate cancer cells." October 2010.*

with heartburn? Well, while spicy food can be a trigger for some people, some studies[4] have shown that capsaicin can actually reduce heartburn symptoms. Capsaicin binds to TRPV1 receptors in the cells of the stomach. This binding action has many potential physiological effects, including increased gastric motility and emptying. When you increase the rate at which the stomach empties during a meal, you prevent it from filling and placing excess pressure on the LES, thereby decreasing reflux.

Licorice

When people refer to taking licorice for heartburn relief, they are usually talking about a herbal supplement rather than candy. In fact, most of the licorice candies you find in the grocery store do not contain licorice extract at all (if they do, it is usually clearly marked on the label). Licorice is marketed as a remedy for a variety of gastrointestinal issues including ulcers, heartburn and gastritis. Like most herbal remedies, there has not been much clinical research to explore the effectiveness of licorice. According to the National Medicines Comprehensive Database[5], licorice has been rated as "possibly effective" for heartburn relief, based on the study of a supplement that included licorice and a variety of other herbs. However, excessive consumption of licorice extract can be toxic. Licorice contains a substance called glycyrrhizic acid, which has been linked to headaches, swelling, sodium retention, loss of potassium and high blood pressure. If you try this home remedy, be sure to go slowly and take it in moderation.

Coconut Oil

Some believe coconut oil suppresses appetite and quickly gives your stomach a feeling of being full. This decreases the desire to ingest more food and encourages consumption of smaller portions at mealtimes. It is well known that overeating can trigger acid reflux. Too much food in the stomach creates pressure, and the pressure forces acid up into the esophagus, resulting in pain and burning sensations. Eating smaller portions is one of the key ways to avoiding acid reflux symptoms. If you want to try coconut oil, substitute the oil that you typically use daily with the same amount of extra-virgin coconut oil. For instance, if a recipe calls for two tablespoons of butter, margarine, vegetable oil or olive oil, simply replace it with an equal amount of coconut oil.

Use Caution and Talk to Your Doctor

As mentioned earlier, there is very little scientific evidence supporting the effectiveness of these home remedies as treatment alternatives for GERD. We encourage you to discuss these with your doctor before you use them to treat your reflux. You never know, you might just find something in your pantry that works for you!

---

[4] *Rodriguez-Stanley S1, Collings KL, Robinson M, Owen W, Miner PB Jr. 1. The Oklahoma Foundation for Digestive Research, University of Oklahoma Health Sciences Center, Oklahoma City, OK 73104, USA. "The effects of capsaicin on reflux, gastric emptying and dyspepsia." January 2014.*
[5] *U.S. National Library of Medicine. "Licorice." Last Reviewed 15 February 2015*

Section II
Four Components of a GERD-Friendly Diet

Introduction
Message From Kimberly A. Tessmer, RDN, LD, Dietitian, Consultant, and Author

"RefluxMD does not rely on medications, but rather digs into the underlying reasons for your condition. This is the only way to control acid reflux for life, and to prevent both the symptoms and the medical issues it can cause in the long term."

As a dietitian, it is hardly unusual for me to hear questions from people concerning acid reflux and GERD. Most of us, including myself, have experienced that uncomfortable fiery sensation in our chests after stuffing ourselves with too much food or eating foods that do not quite agree with our digestive systems. Heartburn caused by acid reflux and GERD is an extremely common problem in the United States, so you are hardly alone. If you suffer from symptoms of acid reflux, then you know firsthand how debilitating it can be. For some people acid reflux occurs occasionally, but for many others it rears its ugly head on a daily basis and eventually becomes GERD.

If you have been diagnosed with GERD, it is time to get the education, help and support you need to control it and get your life back. Avoid falling into the trap of popping OTC or prescription medication every time you eat, just to relieve your impending symptoms. Taking a pill may be much easier, but all it will do is cover up the root cause of your GERD and may potentially cause other health issues. These medications are not meant to be used as a long-term solution for your condition. Your goal should be to find out what is truly causing your acid reflux and to make the changes necessary to free yourself from the troubling symptoms. Potential causes for these symptoms may be anything from food to lifestyle to emotional issues.

RefluxMD is a tool that you can use to assist you through this process. This website, which is staffed by professionally-trained medical advisors, can educate you in what acid reflux and GERD are and what it takes to banish your symptoms once and for all! RefluxMD does not rely on medications, but rather digs into the underlying reasons for your condition. This is the only way to control acid reflux for life, and to prevent both the symptoms and the medical issues it can cause in the long term.

I recently wrote a book entitled *Your Nutrition Solution to Acid Reflux*. My book is aligned with the goals and insights of RefluxMD, so when they asked to me join their advisory board I was thrilled. It was refreshing to find a website that takes a nutritional and lifestyle-based approach to this growing problem. My book and RefluxMD go hand-in-hand with the same type of behavior-changing approach, in terms of food choice and eating habits, smoking, alcohol use, obesity, and other lifestyle habits that tend to be the culprit. I look forward to working with RefluxMD and providing my expertise to help those with acid reflux to suffer no more!

Sincerely,
Kimberly A. Tessmer, RDN, LD

About Kimberly Tessmer RDN, LD

Kimberly Tessmer is a Registered Dietitian Nutritionist and Licensed Dietitian in the State of Ohio as well as a published author. She is the founder and owner of Nutrition Focus, which offers a wide range of nutritional services for individuals online as well as both small and large organizations and businesses. Ms. Tessmer has over twenty years of experience in the field of nutrition and has authored nine books to date with more to come. She holds a Bachelor of Science degree in technology and dietetics from Bowling Green State University in Bowling Green, Ohio. Ms. Tessmer has extensive experience in this area. She worked in hospitals, nursing homes, and as a corporate dietitian for three national weight loss companies before launching Nutrition Focus. You can connect with Ms. Tessmer via Facebook and Twitter, and her books can be purchased from Amazon in various formats.

Section II: Overview

"Diet is critical for everyone with GERD, though many people with acid reflux are not considered overweight or they are happy with their current weight. Therefore, RefluxMD's GERD-friendly diet was designed to apply to everyone, even though the targets and goals of each individual may vary."

Now that you have a good understanding of GERD – its causes, symptoms, potential complications and treatment options – we can get into the "meat and potatoes" (a little GERD diet joke) and purpose for this book. In this section we will delve into one of the most effective treatment options available to GERD sufferers – a GERD-friendly diet. Most physicians recommend dietary changes to their patients with acid reflux because a modified diet can help reduce symptoms and halt the progression of the disease. The goal of RefluxMD's diet plan is to either completely eliminate or noticeably reduce your GERD symptoms.

In this section we will explain in detail the four main components of the RefluxMD GERD-friendly diet, including 1) proper nutrition, 2) portion control, 3) weight management, and 4) avoiding trigger foods. These chapters provide the fundamental conceptual understanding of the diet plan that is necessary before you build your action plan. The following section will detail the step-by-step process for putting this plan into practice.

It is important to note that part of our plan is devoted to weight loss. Excess body weight and GERD have a strong correlation, so this diet plan is designed for anyone seeking to eliminate excess weight. Diet is critical for everyone with GERD, though many people with acid reflux are not considered overweight or they are happy with their current weight. Therefore, RefluxMD's GERD-friendly diet was designed to apply to everyone, even though the targets and goals of each individual may vary. Throughout this book we provide options relevant to those who seek to lose weight, as well as those who aim to maintain their weight.

Chapter 12 – Proper Nutrition

The first key component discussed is modifying dietary patterns to achieve proper nutrition. In this section we focus on things you SHOULD do, whereas much of the management of this disease is about things NOT to do (i.e. avoiding trigger foods, large portions, fatty foods, etc.). The foundations of this chapter are based on one of the most successful diet plans ever created, the DASH diet, which was named "Best Overall Diet" by *U.S. News & World Report* for 2015[6]. Originally created by the National Institutes of Health (NIH), the DASH diet is a well-balanced diet that includes fruits, vegetables,

[6] *U.S. News Staff. "Best Diets 2015." U.S. News & World Report, 6 January 2015.*

fish, low fat dairy, nuts, lean meats, poultry, whole grains, healthy fats and other foods that are rich in beneficial nutrients. The U.S. News & World Report evaluated 35 of the most popular diets with input from a panel of experts. Here is what they had to say about the DASH diet:

> *"Mirroring the federal government's 2010 Dietary Guidelines, the diet came in at No. 1 in this category. The majority of panelists gave it the maximum of 5. Experts called the approach the 'gold standard' and 'nutritionally sound"."*

Chapter 13 – Portion Control

In this chapter we address stomach distension and how it impacts reflux disease to highlight the importance of portion control. There are many different potential causes for stomach distension. We address the three main reasons this occurs: frequent overeating and large portion sizes, prolonged bloating and stomach pressure, and excessive belly weight. In each part of this chapter we discuss why these behaviors, conditions, and triggers can worsen GERD and how you can guard against them.

Chapter 14 – Weight Management

The third component of understanding our reflux diet plan is weight management. As was mentioned earlier, obesity is one of the top risk factors for GERD. Given the current status of the obesity epidemic in this country, many people will need to lose weight if they want to effectively address their acid reflux condition. For those who are not overweight, this chapter includes important tips for maintaining a healthy weight, and we strongly encourage you to read it. In this chapter, we discuss the relationship between BMI and GERD, how to determine your BMI score, and things you can do to reduce that score. In the last part of this chapter we discuss exercise, its role in weight management, and safety concerns regarding these types of activities.

Chapter 15 – Avoiding Trigger Foods

In this chapter we address trigger foods, how to identify them, and how to avoid them. We will help you to create a food journal so you can identify trigger foods that are specific to you. This chapter will help you to find the triggers that cause your symptoms and reinforce a discipline to avoid them. We also examine the harmful effects that alcohol and tobacco use can have on reflux and provide suggestions for curbing those habits.

---

[7] Hiatt, Kurtis. *"DASH Diet Expert Reviews." U.S. News & World Report, 01 December 2012*

Chapter 12
Proper Nutrition

"The DASH diet has assembled an ideal balance of key nutritional elements to provide a healthy eating plan. RefluxMD has taken this plan one step further, by modifying the diet program and eliminating items that are also known to cause GERD symptoms."

A well-balanced and healthy diet is not only essential for a high quality of life, it is a necessity for anyone suffering from acid reflux disease. Regardless of your weight, if you suffer from acid reflux disease, healthy eating is a must.

Over the past few decades, theories and philosophies about the "ideal" diet have undergone many changes. In the 1980s, most diets recommended a high level of carbohydrate consumption and put severe limits on fats. Most popular diet plans followed the nutritional beliefs of the time. After several years, this thinking changed. Carbohydrate consumption was reexamined and soon found that excessive amounts contribute to obesity and higher cholesterol levels. Many in the diet industry were also surprised to find that certain fats consumed in moderation were necessary for good health. If you are confused and unsure of the "right" components that make up a healthy diet, you are not alone.

The DASH Diet
In the first half of the 1990s, The NIH, an agency of the U.S. Department of Health and Human Services, funded research[8] to determine if diet could influence blood pressure, to help address the alarming increase in hypertension among adults. This effort led to the largest and most comprehensive diet research study ever undertaken up to that point. This massive government initiative lasted four years and was conducted by five of the leading health research centers in the country. The results of that research led to what is known as one of the most proven and effective diets ever created, the DASH diet.

Although the DASH diet's primary goal was to lower blood pressure, it would subsequently become the "gold standard" for a well-balanced diet. Since its creation, the DASH diet's proven philosophies have time and again been a life changer for many who have followed its guidelines and principles.

The DASH diet[9] is rich in fruits, vegetables, fat-free or low fat dairy products, whole

---

[8] *National Institute of Health. "Dietary Patterns and Blood Pressure." NIH Guide, Volume 21, Number 36, 9 October 1992*

[9] *National Institute of Health. "What is the DASH Eating Plan?" National Heart, Lung, and Blood Institute. 6 June 2014.*

grains, fish, poultry, beans, seeds and nuts. It also contains less salt and sodium, sweets, added sugars, sugar-containing beverages, saturated fats and red meats. This heart-healthy way of eating is low in saturated fat, trans fat and cholesterol, and rich in nutrient-dense foods that are associated with lowering blood pressure — mainly potassium, magnesium and calcium, as well as protein and fiber. Below we describe several key components of the Dash diet, with explanations for why each is important for good health and how they pertain to the symptoms of acid reflux. In Sections V and VI, you will find recipes rich in the above mentioned nutrients and foods, as well as twenty-one daily eating plans that put all of these concepts into action.

Fiber

Fiber provides many digestive benefits. Studies[10] have indicated that a high-fiber diet can be an effective aid in reducing acid reflux symptoms, by lowering gastric acid levels. Fiber is not digested, but rather is a prebiotic that provides food for beneficial gut bacteria, which helps to boost digestive health. It is also believed to be an effective aid in achieving and maintaining a healthy weight, because foods high in fiber are typically low in calories and help to make you feel fuller longer. Since they linger longer in the stomach, they satisfy your appetite with less calories. Many fiber-rich foods are chewy; as a result, people tend to eat them at a slower pace. Slower eating typically leads to less total food consumption, resulting in smaller meals.

Fiber comes in two forms: soluble (which dissolves in water) and insoluble (which does not dissolve in water). Soluble fiber is believed to help lower LDL cholesterol, or the "bad" kind. Insoluble fiber helps to move food through the digestive system and provides bulk in stools, which can help to keep bowel movements regular. Overall, consuming a fiber-rich diet results in a healthier digestive system. The DASH diet includes many sources of fiber including fruits, vegetables, whole grains, nuts, beans and seeds.

Minerals

Minerals keep us healthy in countless ways. Some minerals are needed in abundance (macrominerals) and others are needed only in small amounts (trace minerals) in order to keep our bodies functioning properly. We will discuss three of the macrominerals found in foods here: potassium, calcium and magnesium.

Potassium plays a vital role in metabolism – regulating sodium levels, transporting nutrients to cells, maintaining hydration of cells, regulating blood pressure and storing energy. Potassium also helps to neutralize stomach acid, and is believed to help protect

---

[10] *Swanson, Kelly. "Dietary fiber alters gut bacteria, supports gastrointestinal health." College of Agriculture Consumer and Environmental Sciences, University of Illinois, Urbana. 27 June 2012.*

against osteoporosis and kidney stones.

Calcium is an essential mineral with the main purpose in the body of building and maintaining bone density. In more recent years, calcium has been found to play a larger role in metabolism than was previously thought. Calcium promotes fat to be burned for energy, as well as aiding the nervous system and muscular function. The recommended daily amount (RDA) of calcium is 1,000-1,200 mg for adults. The daily limit for calcium is 2,000-2,500 mg daily. It is important to stay within these guidelines, for regular overconsumption of this mineral can lead to kidney stones, constipation, impaired absorption of iron and zinc, as well as calcium buildup in the blood vessels.

Magnesium is a mineral that is mainly stored by the body inside bones. It plays a large part in bone metabolism, nervous system function, energy production and blood sugar regulation, and helps to control inflammation. Low magnesium intake may cause acid reflux symptoms. Those suffering from GERD might consider having their doctor check their magnesium levels and question them about the need for a magnesium supplement.

The DASH diet places emphasis on consumption of nutrient-dense foods containing all of these minerals. By emphasizing the consumption of low-fat dairy products such as milk, yogurt, cottage cheese and cheese, a calcium-rich diet may be achieved. Potassium and magnesium are plentiful in whole grains, fruits, vegetables, nuts, beans, seeds and low-fat dairy, and are amply incorporated in the diet as well.

Sodium

Sodium is a chemical element that is necessary for neural brain function. It is essential for controlling blood pressure and blood volume as well as helping muscles and nerves to function properly. Although sodium is essential to good health, too much sodium can lead to high blood pressure, heart failure, osteoporosis, kidney disease, stomach cancer and an increased risk of stroke over time. In fact, the NIH states that one in three adults suffer from hypertension[11], the leading cause of strokes and coronary heart disease. Scientific research has mainly focused on hypertension prevention and management by reduced sodium consumption. In fact, the NIH reported[12] in the results of a multi-center clinical trial that dietary salt reduction, weight loss, or both in combination, reduced blood pressure in patients with hypertension and decreased their need for medication.

Sodium levels may play a role in GERD symptoms as well. A study[13] in Sweden found that adults who "always salted their food were seventy percent more likely to

[11] *National Institute of Health. "What is High Blood Pressure?" 2 August 2012*

[12] *National Institute of Health. "Statement on Sodium Intake and High Blood Pressure." 17 August 1998.*

[13] *Yael Waknine. Smoking, High Salt Intake May Be Risk Factors for Acid Reflux. Medscape. Nov 11, 2004.*

suffer from acid reflux compared with those who never added salt." However, sodium intake goes beyond the saltshaker because sodium saturates many processed meats and canned foods. The DASH diet is a low-sodium plan that avoids processed foods, and encourages the consumption of fresh whole foods in their natural form.

Healthy Fats

In 2004, the U.S. Food and Drug Administration announced a "qualified health claim[14]" that omega-3 fatty acids were a healthy beneficial nutrient. Although fats were never strictly limited by the diet and were generally understood as a necessary energy source by nutritionists, most early diet plans placed significant limitations on their consumption. The DASH diet embraces healthy fats as an important part of a balanced diet. Healthy fats are important for many reasons, including cellular construction, oxygen and vitamin transportation, assisting brain and nerve function, aiding healthy blood clotting, providing body insulation and keeping skin soft. Monounsaturated fats and polyunsaturated fats are considered "healthy." Consuming controlled amounts of each can help to reduce the risk of heart disease, regulate insulin levels and assist in lowering LDL cholesterol levels.

Omega-3 fatty acids are a form of polyunsaturated fat that has been shown in research studies[15] to aid in cognitive development in infants, play a role in mood stability, help in the treatment of depression, and play a key role in heart health. It should be noted that the best form of omega-3 fatty acids are those found in fatty fish such as salmon, mackerel, herring, trout and tuna. People often take these healthy fats as a supplement in the form of fish oil capsules. These supplements can cause reflux episodes for some people, so those with acid reflux disease may want to avoid them. These healthy fats can also be found in certain nuts and avocados, both of which all are incorporated into the DASH diet.

Unhealthy Fats

The DASH diet places strict limitations on unhealthy fats, trans fats and saturated fats by emphasizing consumption of lean meats, fish, skinless poultry, and low-fat dairy. Like sodium, these unhealthy fats can increase the risk of heart disease and stroke as well as other health issues. These fats are also a known trigger for acid reflux and can contribute to obesity, another cause of GERD.

Protein

The DASH diet does not shy away from protein, but emphasizes lower fat options such as skinless poultry, fish/seafood and lean red meats as the primary sources. Protein

[14] U.S. Department of Health & Human Services. "FDA Announces Qualified Health Claims for Omega-3 Fatty Acids." 8 September 2004.

[15] National Center for Complementary and Integrative Health. Omega-3 Supplements: An Introduction. July 2009.

is an essential building block for muscles, tissue repair, immunity support, hormone and enzyme creation, and it provides a great source of energy. Protein is a nutrient that breaks down slowly in the digestive process, and thus tends to satisfy hunger for a longer period of time than other foods. Unfortunately, the breakdown of protein requires an increased level of stomach acid, which is something those with GERD would ideally like to avoid. The solution is to consume a moderate amount of protein daily. On the positive side, meals with a higher protein ratio produce less stomach distension, because stomach bacteria do not multiply to the same degree in which they typically do when digesting carbohydrates and sugars. Protein is also found in nuts, beans, lentils and soy-based foods.

Carbohydrates

The DASH diet is not considered a low-carbohydrate diet, rather, it focuses on managing the amount of carbohydrates consumed. The DASH diet recommends eating healthier whole grains instead of refined carbohydrates, in order to reduce the levels of sugar and nutrient-devoid calories in the diet. Carbohydrate consumption is encouraged in the form of fruits, vegetables, whole grains, beans and other healthy sources. There is growing support[16] for the concept that excessive consumption of carbohydrates adversely impacts the balance of healthy bacteria in the digestive system, which may cause abdominal and stomach disruption as well as acid reflux symptoms.

Vitamins and the Benefits of Antioxidants

Vitamins are essential for cellular maintenance, development and growth. A well-balanced diet like the DASH diet provides more than ample amounts of vitamins needed by most adults on a daily basis. Various types of nutrients, including vitamins, minerals and phytochemicals have antioxidant properties and act as antioxidants in the body. Antioxidants defend cells against what are known as free radicals, which are created naturally in the body and may also result from exposure to environmental hazards such as smoking and pollution. Free radicals pose a threat to healthy cells that can lead to cancer and other health issues. Healthy nutritional programs like the DASH diet can reduce the production of free radicals and promote the consumption of antioxidants to ensure good cellular health. Antioxidant consumption is promoted by the DASH diet in the form of fruit, vegetables, beans and certain vitamin-E rich nuts such as almonds.

Calories

Calories are a unit of measurement used to describe the amount of energy in a given food. Any food that provides energy to our bodies can be measured in calories. In theory, if you burn the same amount of calories that you consume, you should maintain

---

[16] *Kresser, Chris. "The hidden causes of heartburn and GERD." ChrisKresser.com 1 April 2010*

your weight. If you consume less energy (calories) than you burn, you will lose weight; conversely, you will gain weight if you consume more calories than you use. One important goal of the DASH diet is to help you to determine the correct amount of calories to consume on a daily and weekly basis, by using age, gender and physical activity levels to estimate calorie needs.

The DASH Diet: An Ideal Balance

Overall, the DASH diet has assembled an ideal balance of key nutritional elements to provide a healthy eating plan. It recommends consuming foods that contain ample amounts of key nutrients and limits potentially harmful or nutrient-devoid foods. RefluxMD has taken this plan one step further by modifying the diet program and eliminating items that are also known to cause GERD symptoms. Based on this foundation, the following sections put these principles into action, providing advice for creating your diet plan and offering a wide variety of delicious GERD-appropriate recipes.

Chapter 13
Portion Control

"Infrequent stomach distension does not cause acid reflux. However, a long period of sustained stomach distension can be the underlying cause of GERD."

How overfilling the stomach caused acid reflux

Stomach distension occurs when the abdomen expands well beyond its normal resting state. In this section we will describe the diet and lifestyle triggers that may cause longer and more sustained periods of stomach distension, which has proven to be a major cause of acid reflux.

To be clear, infrequent stomach distension does not cause acid reflux. However, a long period of sustained stomach distension can be the underlying cause of GERD. The main connection between stomach distension and acid reflux is the harmful effect it has on the lower esophageal sphincter (LES). As discussed in Section I, the LES is a valve-like muscle that exists at the junction of the stomach and the esophagus. The LES opens to let foods pass and closes to keep stomach contents from rising upward, except when vomiting or burping.

Any time the stomach expands, the LES stretches. The LES is durable and can withstand a considerable amount of stretching, but extreme prolonged and sustained abdomen expansion can gradually diminish LES function. A good way to describe the impact of stomach distension is to use a balloon as an example. Imagine a rubber balloon that is fifty percent inflated. The inflated section is your stomach and the neck of the balloon is your esophagus. The LES is at the junction of these two parts of the balloon. Imagine that you used a black marker to circle the LES on the balloon. What do you think will happen to that black circle when you blow more air into the balloon? Of course, the black circle will expand and be pulled toward the inflated part of the balloon.

This mirrors what happens to your LES when your stomach is distended. As in our balloon example, when the stomach is repeatedly distended, the muscle is stretched. Over time, the muscle begins to lose its barrier function. For example, the more frequently you overeat, the more likely it is that your LES muscle may lose strength over time and become shorter in length. Eventually, the LES could lose its effectiveness as a barrier completely. Years of excessive pulling and widening of the LES can severely weaken it, which can lead to chronic GERD. The main causes of stomach distension that cause damage to the LES are frequent overeating and large portion sizes, prolonged bloating and stomach pressure, and excessive belly weight.

Implications of Overeating

Overeating is widespread in economically developed nations where food is readily available at reasonable prices. It should be of no surprise that these same countries have the highest rates of GERD. The link between the two is clear: with affluence comes excessive behavior, including gluttony. Essentially, when an abundance of high-quality foods are available, people tend to eat for enjoyment rather than consume it for basic survival. For many in economically developed nations, overindulgence is a prevalent temptation. Likewise, in less developed and poorer nations, where food is far less abundant, the incidence of GERD is substantially less[17].

Eating a large meal that pushes your stomach beyond normal capacity stretches the LES and causes increased upward internal pressure. That pressure can force stomach contents to move upward, causing regurgitation. Anyone who has overeaten at a Thanksgiving dinner has most likely experienced an episode of regurgitation not long after finishing his or her meal. When people do this habitually at most meals over many years, damage and weakness to the LES can grow so bad that any meal, regardless of size, can regurgitate up into the esophagus and cause symptoms of acid reflux.

Overeating can also cause the stomach to produce more acid in order to fully digest the massive amount of food. In addition, larger meals take longer to digest, which can significantly increase the amount of time that food and acid remain in the stomach. For those who regularly overeat, everyday actions such as bending over or lying down may result in regurgitation.

Limiting portion sizes may help to prevent regurgitation and the progression of GERD. Those who suffer from this disease should eat less at each meal and manage their portion sizes with diligence. The idea is to listen to your body and eat until you are comfortable, not stuffed. This requires planning for smaller meals by adding healthy snacks during the day to fend off hunger.

Reducing Portion Size and Snacking

Reducing the size of your meals will aid digestion and put less pressure on your LES. Reduced portions can be advantageous for anyone suffering from GERD because they take less time to digest, they create less abdominal pressure, and less stomach acid is required for digestion.

Given these facts, it is highly advisable to eat five to six smaller meals per day instead of the traditional three meals of breakfast, lunch and dinner. With five meals, calorie

---

[17] *Jansson C1, Wallander MA, Johansson S, Johnsen R, Hveem K. Upper Gastrointestinal Research, Department of Molecular Medicine and Surgery, Karolinska Institutet, Stockholm, Sweden. "Stressful psychosocial factors and symptoms of gastroesophageal reflux disease: a population-based study in Norway." 2010*

content can be maintained by reducing the size of each meal. There are several simple tricks you can incorporate in your diet plan that will not require major changes to your current routine. For example, instead of eating eggs, ham, potatoes and toast for breakfast, try having ham and eggs alone and eliminate the potatoes and toast. You can trade the potatoes and toast for a quick mid-morning snack, or try a small bowl of high-fiber cereal instead. Rather than choosing a twelve-inch submarine sandwich for lunch, switch to a six-inch or eight-inch size, avoid the chips and drink water in place of soft drinks. This is an easy first step towards changing your diet: reduce the size of what you already eat in your three main courses, and spread the same number of calories over an increased number of smaller, more frequent meals.

Next, begin to incorporate some snacks after you have reduced the size of each meal. Nuts and fruits are quick and easy, and they are satiating between meals. These snacks may add some incremental calories, but they may reduce your total daily calorie intake as a whole if you manage your meal choices and portions. Snacking has another important objective: it keeps you from feeling hungry in between meals, which can lead to overindulging. Effectively managing your appetite between meals is an important part of staying on your meal plan, and can help you to feel satisfied with smaller portions at main meals. Too many diet plans simply reduce the size of the three main meals, resulting in extreme hunger in between meals. These plans are destined to fail. To keep yourself from falling off your meal plan with reduced main meal sizes, be sure to incorporate healthy snacks in between meals.

Curbing Carbonation, Gas, and Bloating

Certain foods and carbonated drinks that cause bloating and gas can also distend the stomach and negatively impact the LES. Increased intra-abdominal pressure caused by gas and bloating can stretch the LES and may permanently impair its function over time. Furthermore, excessive air and pressure in the stomach can increase the propensity to belch, exposing the esophagus to potentially harmful stomach acid. Maintaining a diet that avoids bloat-causing foods and carbonated drinks is an important part of an effective reflux diet.

Carbonated Drinks

Many people find carbonated drinks to be tasty, and a large part of their appeal is the carbonation itself. The bubbly fizz of soda pop gives off a thirst-quenching sensation, followed by a relieving belch that people have found irresistible for decades. However, times have changed. Fifty years ago access to soft drinks was limited, and as a consequence they were considered an occasional treat or perhaps an after-meal dessert. Today, soft drinks make up a major portion of many people's daily fluid intake. It is not unusual to find adults who drink four or more carbonated drinks a day.

A study done in 2011 by the National Center for Health Statistics[18] found that Americans get 8% of daily calories from sugary drinks. In an article by CNN about this study, they commented on the widespread prevalence of soda pop in modern day America.

> *"When it was first invented, soda pop was a treat most people had once in a while for special occasions.*
>
> *Now it's a daily fixture in American life -- in bright containers glowing inside vending machines, chugged from 32-ounce bucket-like containers at self-service stations and served as the default beverage in fast-food meals."*

According to a Gallup poll in July 2012[19], 48% of Americans reported drinking at least one glass of soda per day (the other 52% say they normally drink no soda). From the 1970s until today, the amount consumed by youths between the ages of 6 and 17 has risen from 56% from 37%[20]. Consequently, this dramatic increase in soda has lead to a larger intake in sugar, a major contributor to obesity.

Simply stated, carbonated drinks cause your stomach to distend to a greater degree than do non-carbonated drinks. One of the best recommendations for avoiding stomach distension is to significantly reduce or eliminate consumption of all carbonated drinks.

Foods that Cause Gas and Bloating

Many people find that certain carbohydrates are a trigger for gas and bloating. For some years, diets low in carbohydrates have been popular solutions for weight loss. Although these diets have recently come under scrutiny based on the latest nutritional research (and new interpretations of past research), they have oftentimes resulted in one very interesting benefit: stomach pressure relief. Further theories[21] suggest that a low-carbohydrate diet can reduce incidences of gut bacterial overgrowth, which may relieve intra-abdominal pressure as an associated positive side effect.

Bacterial Overgrowth and Carbohydrates

Proper digestion requires an ample amount of stomach acid to break down the molecular structure of food. When the stomach does not secrete the necessary amount of gastric acid needed for proper digestion, a portion of the contents remain in the stomach, providing a rich environment for potentially harmful stomach bacteria.

[18] *Ogden CL, Kit BK, Carroll MD, Park S. Consumption of sugar drinks in the United States, 2005–2008. NCHS data brief, no 71. Hyattsville, MD: National Center for Health Statistics. 2011.*

[19] *Saad, Lydia. "Nearly Half of Americans Drink Soda Daily." Gallup. 23 July 2012*

[20] *Park, Madison. "Half of Americans sip sugary drinks daily." CNN. 31 August 2011.*

[21] *Kresser, Chris. "The hidden causes of heartburn and GERD." Chris Kresser 1 April 2010*

In combination with partially digested or undigested food, this bacteria produces a fermentation process that creates stomach gas, resulting in increased intra-abdominal pressure. The stomach bacteria then multiply, and bacterial overgrowth leads to more intense gas and bloating. Highly refined and processed or "unhealthy" carbohydrates (such as white bread, pasta and white rice, to name a few) provide an easy molecular structure for stomach bacteria to break down. Because they provide more easily accessible food for the bacteria, they tend to produce higher levels of fermentation and greater amounts of stomach gas. "Healthy" carbohydrates (whole grains and starchy vegetables, for example) have the opposite effect. Unhealthy highly refined carbohydrates should be avoided and healthier whole grains should be consumed to promote healthy bacterial flora in the intestines.

Probiotics to Regulate Bacterial Overgrowth

Probiotics are microorganisms that live in the digestive tract. They are a form of bacteria and are considered "good" because they help to strengthen the immune system, assist in digestion and work as agents to improve overall health. Probiotics help to reduce harmful bacteria by competing with them for resources. This competition helps to limit the growth of harmful bacteria, and a balance is achieved with the reduction of potentially harmful bacterial overgrowth. With bacterial overgrowth under control, less bacterial fermentation occurs, ultimately reducing intra-abdominal pressure and resulting in fewer reflux episodes. Yogurt and other fermented foods contain live and active cultures as a good source of probiotics, and fiber has been known to aid the growth of "good" bacteria as well.

Fat and Other Causes

Dietary fat can cause stomach distension, which leads to gas and bloating. Food that is high in fat requires more time to digest, and may result in a bloated feeling. Since fat requires more time to digest, the stomach empties more slowly and signals a need for more acid to break down its large molecular structure.

Bloating may also occur after eating too fast, after smoking, during periods of high stress and after excessive alcohol consumption. It is important to keep an eye out for any foods that can cause the development of excess gas. Everyone is different, and those with this problem should keep a list of the foods, beverages, and ingredients that may cause bloating and gas.

Belly Weight Can Also Be a Factor

Excessive weight in the midriff section (abdomen) is believed to be another potential underlying cause of acid reflux. The association between overeating and excessive intra-abdominal pressure is well documented[22]. Furthermore, a sagging overweight belly is believed to be another factor that may compromise the LES, and over time this too can permanently damage the muscle.

Due to the persistent pull of gravity, excess body fat stored in the stomach area has a tendency to drag the stomach downward and stretch it beyond its natural extension. With this consistent downward pressure the LES also becomes affected, as it is stretched to provide necessary slack for the stomach. With enough time and pressure, the LES can become permanently slack and remain open, providing a gateway for upward-flowing gastric acids.

Diet and Belly Weight

Eating healthily can have a strong impact on body weight. The DASH diet, outlined in Chapter 12 of this section, provides dietary suggestions for anyone looking to lose weight. The action plan required to implement this diet will be detailed in section three. The DASH diet was developed to control caloric intake, reduce fat consumption, increase fiber intake, and encourage consumption of other fat-fighting minerals such as calcium. A healthy diet is your friend in the battle against excessive weight, including extra belly fat.

Exercise and Belly Fat

There are two types of exercises that can help to reduce weight and may also impact belly weight. One type is the cardiovascular workout, comprised of exercises that increase heart rate and keep it at higher levels for a period of time. Repetitive and consistent cardiovascular workouts might include jogging, swimming, elliptical training and walking at a brisk pace. Regular exercise will begin to burn calories, and fat will begin to disappear over time when paired with a healthy diet.

Other activities to reduce excess fat that may have more impact on the midsection include direct abdomen exercises, which are designed to increase and strengthen the abdominal muscles. Many who embark on this type of exercise program may become frustrated because an unyielding layer of fat perpetually remains on top of a stronger and larger set of muscles. Even though these types of exercises may not yield immediate results or a "beach-body" look, stronger abdominal muscles will result in less stomach sag and less pressure on the LES.

For those with an "inner tube"-sized layer of fat around the abdomen, significant time and effort will be required to achieve results. Many have succeeded in reducing their weight and reducing belly fat by working with personal trainers and setting realistic and

---

[22] *Richter, Joel E. Journal for Clinical Gastroenterology and Hepatology. "Advances in GERD." Gatro Hep Advance. Feb 2010.*

achievable waistline goals. Before beginning any exercise program, it is wise to consult your doctor about your diet and exercise plans. Most physicians will make certain that your overall health can support your goals and provide you with additional ideas for reaching your goals in as healthy a way as possible.

Chapter 14
Weight Management

"Overall, epidemiological data shows that maintaining a normal BMI may reduce the likelihood of developing GERD and its potential complications." - Dr. Hashem El-Serag

Reduce Your BMI to Manage Your GERD Symptoms

All GERD specialists encourage their patients to manage three aspects of their lifestyle to reduce GERD symptoms: exercise, weight management and diet. Many physicians use Body Mass Index (BMI) as a tool to determine the risk level of their patients, and the urgency of weight management. Our goal in this chapter is to explain the impact that excessive weight has on GERD, as well as its symptoms and patterns of progression, and to present a rational and safe approach to managing weight.

What is Body Mass Index?

Body Mass Index (BMI) is a number that is calculated based on each individual's height and weight. It has proven to be a useful tool as an indicator of risk associated with several diseases, including type-2 diabetes, high blood pressure, heart disease, and certain cancers. BMI is not a perfect tool, but it is easy to understand and simple to use and interpret. The chart on the next page illustrates the BMI score for a range of heights (from 4'10" to 6'3") and weights (from 100 to 248 pounds). To determine you BMI, simply find your height in blue in the first column, and read across until you find your weight. Then find the red number in the top row to indicate your BMI. For a more accurate BMI calculation, please visit the NIH website to access their BMI calculator.

What does the BMI score mean?

The value of the number is a reasonably good indicator of obesity using the following scale:

Normal weight relative to height: BMI of 18.5 to 24.9
Overweight relative to height: BMI of 25.0 to 29.9
Obese relative to height: BMI of 30 or higher

In general, the goal is to achieve a BMI of less than 25; however, a BMI of 18.5 or less is considered underweight. For anyone attempting to lose weight to reach a lower BMI target, even small losses (between five and ten percent) can be valuable. According to NIH[23] guidelines, those at risk of developing more serious health complications include anyone with a BMI of 30 or more, as well as those with a BMI between 25 and 29.9 in combination with any of the following risk factors:

---

[23] *NIH News. "NIH study identifies ideal body mass index." December 2010.*

- High blood pressure (hypertension)

- High LDL cholesterol ("bad" cholesterol)

- Low HDL cholesterol ("good" cholesterol)

- High triglycerides

- High blood glucose (blood sugar)

- Family history of early heart disease

- Physical inactivity

- Smoking

BMI Chart

BMI	21	22	23	24	25	26	27	28	29	30	31
4'10"	100	105	110	115	119	124	129	134	138	143	148
4'11"	104	109	114	119	124	128	133	138	143	148	153
5'0"	107	112	118	123	128	133	138	143	148	153	158
5'1"	111	116	122	127	132	137	143	148	153	158	164
5'2"	115	120	126	131	136	142	147	153	158	164	169
5'3"	118	124	130	135	141	146	152	158	163	169	175
5'4"	122	128	134	140	145	151	157	163	169	174	180
5'5"	126	132	138	144	150	156	162	168	174	180	186
5'6"	130	136	142	148	155	161	167	173	179	186	192
5'7"	134	140	146	153	159	166	172	178	185	191	198
5'8"	138	144	151	158	164	171	177	184	190	197	203
5'9"	142	149	155	162	169	176	182	189	196	203	209
5'10"	146	153	160	167	174	181	188	195	202	209	216
5'11"	150	157	165	172	179	186	193	200	208	215	222
6'0"	154	162	169	177	184	191	199	206	213	221	228
6'1"	159	166	174	182	189	197	204	212	219	227	235
6'2"	163	171	179	186	194	202	210	218	225	233	241
6'3"	168	176	184	192	200	208	216	224	232	240	248

Obesity and GERD

In September 2008, *Digestive Disease and Sciences* published an article titled "The Association between Obesity and GERD: a Review of the Epidemiological Evidence" by Dr. Hashem El-Serag that analyzed the results of previous research studies on the subject. El-Serag was interested in the relationship between obesity and several GERD-related conditions including esophageal cancer (adenocarcinoma), Barrett's esophagus, esophageal erosion and general GERD symptoms.

According to this review, any increase in weight has the potential to aggravate GERD symptoms, regardless of BMI. This supports the theory that increasing BMI or gaining weight is related to increased prevalence or severity of GERD symptoms. El-Serag concluded, "Overall, epidemiological data shows that maintaining a normal BMI may reduce the likelihood of developing GERD and its potential complications."

RefluxMD's medical director, Dr. William Dengler, authored an article on this subject titled "A Heavy Burden: GERD and Obesity." Dr. Dengler noted that BMI is the measurement of obesity that is most commonly used by physicians, and excellent justification is evidenced for its use. According to Dr. Dengler, "Because of the increase in body mass, obese patients tend to experience a 'squeeze phenomenon' that can force stomach juices upward through the lower esophageal sphincter into the esophagus." He also noted several interesting facts concerning BMI and GERD/GERD symptoms:

- 5-10% of people with a BMI of less than 25 have heartburn less than once a week.

- 20-25% of people with BMI greater than 30 have heartburn more than once a week.

- When tested for GERD via pH study, almost 70% of people with a BMI over 30 tested positive for GERD.

Slow and Steady When it Comes to Weight Loss

Taking your time to lose weight is important, because slow and steady weight loss programs have been shown to be more successful. According to the Centers for Disease Control and Prevention (CDC)[24], a consistent rate of weight loss at one to two pounds per week is ideal, whereas potential complications are associated with more rapid weight loss. A study published by *The American Journal of Medicine*[25] found a consistent statistical relationship between gallstone formation and the rate of weight loss. Their conclusion: "Risk of gallstone formation in obese persons during active weight loss seems to increase in an exponential fashion. The data suggests that rates of weight loss should not exceed an average of 1.5 kg per week (3.3 pounds per week)." So, take it slow.

Setting Goals: Plan your Work and Work your Plan

With a goal of losing two pounds per week, let us explore how to build an effective weight management plan. Meet Robert, who is 5'9" and weighs 196 pounds. Most of his excess weight was gained over the last five years and came with increasing GERD

---

[24] *Center for Disease Control and Prevention. "Losing Weight - What is healthy weight loss?" 17 August 2011.*

[25] *The American Journal of Medicine. MD, DrPH Roland L. Weinsier, MD Louis J. Wilson, PhD Jeannette Lee. "Medically safe rate of weight loss for the treatment of obesity: A guideline based on risk of gallstone formation." 9 May 1994.*

symptoms. According to the chart above, Robert's BMI is 29, which is at the upper end of the overweight range, nearing obese.

With his twenty-year high school reunion scheduled for June 15th, Robert would like to not only look great for his classmates but feel good, too, as he celebrates. But can he do this safely and hit his BMI goal of 25? Again, using the chart above, we can see that a BMI of 25 indicates a target weight of 169 pounds. That equals a targeted weight loss of 27 pounds. If Robert loses two pounds every week, he can lose all 27 pounds in 14 weeks with the right diet changes and increased exercise.

Robert plans to research diet programs, and consult with his physician before beginning his diet on February 1st. Since consistency is not one of his best qualities, he is also planning on the possibility for some "slippage," so he is adding three weeks to his plan – or one "setback week" for every four weeks of successful dieting. The following chart shows Robert's weight loss strategy for meeting his goals in time for the reunion (assumes four weeks in each month):

Target Weight at the Beginning of Each Week

	FEB	MAR	APR	MAY	JUN
Week 1	196	190*	182	176*	170
Week 2	194	188	182*	174	**168**
Week 3	192	186	180	174	
Week 4	190	184	178	172	

* Setback week

For Robert to achieve his goal at a safe pace, with greater potential for maintaining the weight loss, his plan will be carried out in a gradual and steady manner.

The DASH Diet and BMI

With a diet plan rich in fruits, vegetables, lean meats, whole grains and fiber, combined with lower calorie consumption, reduced fat and less sodium, losing weight should be a natural outcome. In essence, this is the exact design behind the DASH diet. If the DASH diet is followed closely, calorie consumption will naturally be reduced, leading to weight reduction. According to the NIH, one pound equals 3500 calories. Therefore, one must either cut 500 calories out of his/her normal diet every day, or burn 500 calories more per day via exercise while maintaining calorie intake, in order to lose one pound per week. It is recommended to first determine how many calories you consume on average every day in order to get a good starting point (more on this in Section III). The reason for this is that blindly launching yourself into a diet plan may result in cutting too many calories at once, which could result in a shock to your system. Below is the recommended daily caloric intake for different types of people, based on age, gender and level of physical activity.

The DASH diet is high in fiber, which alleviates hunger and can help to make a lower-calorie diet more tolerable. When fiber is added to a diet, most people will eat the same amount of food by weight as before while consuming fewer calories. As mentioned earlier, fiber has also been shown to slow down the pace of meals. Due to its tougher texture, fiber typically requires more chewing with each bite, allowing the brain more time to recognize a feeling of fullness. For many, this helps to curtail the urge for unneeded extra helpings. Furthermore, chewing stimulates the production of saliva and stomach juices, which can aid in acid reflux relief.

Estimated Calorie Requirements for Each Gender and Age Group at Three Physical Activity Levels

Gender	Age (years)	Sedentary Lifestyle	Moderately Active Lifestyle	Active Lifestyle
Child	2-3	1,000	1,000-1,400	1,000-1,400
Female	4-8	1,200	1,400-1,600	1,400-1,800
	9-13	1,600	1,600-2,000	1,800-2,200
	14-18	1,800	2,000	2,400
	19-30	2,000	2,000-2,200	2,400
	31-50	1,800	2,000	2,200
	> 50	1,600	1,800	2,000-2,200
Male	4-8	1,400	1,400-1,600	1,600-2,000
	9-13	1,800	1,800-2,200	2,000-2,600
	14-18	2,200	2,400-2,800	2,800-3,200
	19-30	2,400	2,600-2,800	3,000
	31-50	2,200	2,400-2,600	2,800-3,000
	> 50	2,000	2,200-2,400	2,400-2,800

From http://healthpluscoach.files.wordpress.com/2013/11/calorie-allowance2.gif

Exercising and BMI
What is the role of exercise in the treatment for acid reflux?

Either consuming fewer calories or burning more calories than are consumed should result in weight loss. Calories burn naturally, even when we are doing nothing, but exercise burns calories at a much higher rate. Thus, exercise is a critical part of any weight loss program. Combining the DASH diet with regular exercise includes both of these essential components for weight loss -- reducing calorie intake and increasing the amount of calories burned. Most structured weight loss plans start with light exercise, such as walking and lifting light weights, with gradual increases in intensity. Be sure to check with your doctor to make sure your medical condition allows for these types of activities.

Along with weight loss and acid reflux relief, the NIH outlines[26] several other potential benefits of committing to an exercise plan:

- Lowers the risk of heart disease, diabetes, and cancers of the breast, uterus and colon

- Strengthens lungs and helps them to work more efficiently

- Strengthens muscles and helps to maintain joint health

- May slow bone loss

- Results in a feeling of increased energy

- Improves one's ability to relax and cope with stress

- Builds confidence

- Improves ability to fall asleep more quickly and sleep more soundly

- Provides an enjoyable way to share time with friends and family

The NIH also recommends thirty minutes of moderate physical activity be performed most days of the week for improved overall health. For weight maintenance, the NIH recommends sixty minutes of "moderate to vigorous" exercise most days of the week. For those looking to lose weight, the NIH recommends sixty to ninety minutes of moderate physical activity daily.

These exercises can be broken up into intervals, such as fifteen minutes at a time. The NIH cautions those who have not been physically active to start slowly with gradual increases in intensity. A simple ten-minute walk is a fine place to start, gradually walking faster and for longer periods with time.

---

[26] *National Institute of Health. "Aim for a healthy weight - facts about healthy weight." National Heart, Lung and Blood Institute.*

Chapter 15
Avoiding Trigger Foods

"Long-term management of symptoms may be within your own control. Your treatment begins with identifying the foods and activities that contribute to your acid reflux, and avoiding those triggers altogether."

Triggers: Foods and Behaviors That Cause Reflux Episodes

> *"I had this small pain that started near the top of my stomach and then seemed to increase as it radiated up the length of my chest behind my breastbone. I thought I was having a heart attack and called 911. I was both relieved and embarrassed to find out my heart was fine, and that I had severe heartburn."*

The pain caused by GERD can range from a mild dullness or a frequent cough to an overwhelming and debilitating sensation. Unfortunately, as the disease progresses, the discomfort caused by reflux disease can be very disruptive to daily life. Instead of finding the source of the problem, the first instinct of many sufferers is to take medication to address their symptoms. A bottle of antacid tablets or a more potent prescription remedy is often the first line of defense against acid reflux. For many, these medications initially manage their symptoms, so they believe they have found a "cure." However, many experience the return of symptoms months or years later because the cause of their symptoms has never been addressed correctly. There is a healthier alternative to these medications, especially for those in the early stages of reflux disease, and it begins with identifying the foods, beverages, times of day and behaviors that trigger acid reflux.

If you are not already aware of your own GERD triggers, an important first step for you is to identify them. Trial and error is a quick and simple way to do this, and your symptoms will not be reluctant about letting you know which of your dietary habits and behaviors give you discomfort. Although some trigger foods are more common than others, keep in mind that not everyone is the same, and what seems to work for others may not work for you.

Unfortunately, there is no real way to predict what will cause symptoms until they actually occur, so it is a good idea to keep track of what you are consuming, when and how much. Maintaining a diet log is a good way to do this, allowing you to easily reference the foods you consumed prior to an episode of reflux. However, what you eat and drink might not be the only factors contributing to your symptoms. How you consume your meals and what you do immediately after can also play an important role. For example, eating large meals forces your digestive system to work harder, producing more potentially irritating stomach acid in the process. Exercising after a meal, eating before bedtime, lying down after a meal or assuming other bodily positions that assist the reverse flow of digestive enzymes can also trigger symptoms for many people.

Behaviors That Are Known to Trigger Reflux
Eating Large Meals

Portion control is a key element of a GERD-friendly diet. No matter what you eat, if you eat too much in one sitting you can trigger acid reflux symptoms. Large portions stretch your lower esophageal sphincter (LES), reducing its barrier function. Frequent large meals can continue to damage the LES until it completely loses its ability to stop food from flowing back up into the esophagus.

Exercising After a Meal

If you exercise, it is best to do so before a meal, or a few hours after a meal. Exercise can put undue pressure on the diaphragm, thus impacting the LES. This pressure can drive the stomach contents up into the esophagus, resulting in GERD symptoms.

Lying Down After a Meal

For those with a compromised LES, gravity is your friend. Gravity will keep the stomach contents in the stomach as long as you are sitting or standing. However, gravity does not have this effect in a reclined or prone position, and stomach contents may easily flow from the stomach back up into the esophagus.

Eating Close to Bedtime

The digestive process is long, taking up to twenty-four hours and sometimes more. However, the initial phase is a breakdown of proteins that occurs using larger than normal amounts of hydrochloric acid produced by the stomach. Based upon the size of a meal and the meal's contents, it can take from one to several hours before the resulting mixture passes into the small intestine. To minimize or avoid GERD symptoms, it is best to eat meals at least three hours before bedtime. Water and easy-to-digest light snacks are acceptable (avoid trigger foods and caffeine) if necessary.

Smoking

A link between GERD symptoms and smoking has been confirmed by research[27]. There are several issues concerning the smoke from tobacco. First, the nicotine is believed to relax the LES, thus reducing the muscle's barrier capabilities. Second, it is believed that smoking results in the production of less saliva, a natural substance that reduces stomach acid and coats the esophagus.

---

[27] *Queensland Institute of Medical Research. "Interactions among smoking, obesity, and symptoms of acid reflux in Barrett's esophagus." Nov 2005.*

Common Foods and Beverages That Trigger GERD Symptoms

As mentioned previously, everyone is different, and may not react the same way to each of these items. However, this list of common triggers should help you to create a "trial and error" program to identify what causes your symptoms.

- Carbonated beverages

- Chocolate

- Citrus fruits

- Drinks or foods that contain caffeine

- Garlic and onions

- Mint

- Spicy foods

- Fatty or fried foods

- Tomatoes and tomato-based foods

There is an additional item that must be mentioned – alcohol. Alcohol is widely consumed and is often associated with social enjoyment. However, for those suffering from acid reflux disease, alcohol should be avoided. We address both smoking and alcohol again in this chapter.

Long-term management of symptoms may be within your own control. Your treatment begins with identifying the foods and activities that contribute to your acid reflux, and avoiding those triggers altogether.

Keeping a Food Journal

A set list of common trigger foods is well accepted by GERD experts, but identifying your trigger foods and then managing your diet accordingly can be a challenge. To succeed, you will need the appropriate tools to identify the foods and behaviors that trigger your acid reflux symptoms, and then build a plan to eliminate them from your diet. With some work and attention to detail, you will find that you can often successfully avoid heartburn and other symptoms that result from GERD.

Find Which Journal Works for You

We have designed two different ways for you to "journal" your dietary intake and symptom history. The first is a simple food journal that will capture a minimum amount of data and effectively identify your trigger foods. The second model is a more comprehensive approach, incorporating several additional factors to identify the underlying causes of your GERD symptoms. Ideally, everyone would choose the second plan because we think it is more effective, but some may see it as too time consuming. The first option is simple and may be maintained while "on the run." We encourage you to evaluate both journal options and choose the one that will work best for you.

Both journal options are available to download and print from our website. After reading this chapter, please see http://www.refluxmd.com/gerd-diet-forms and print the option that best suits you.

Option 1: Simple Food Journal

The end goal of your food journal is to identify the foods and behaviors that are triggering your reflux episodes. This food journal model attempts to achieve this goal in the simplest possible way. This is not a daily or weekly journal, and has no set time frame for completing journal entries. With this method, you are only required to keep a record after a symptom or episode occurs.

Trigger Foods

First, identify what you ate in your last meal that may have contributed to your symptoms. If there were specific ingredients that were part of, or combined with, the foods – like raw onions or tomato eaten with a hamburger – you must include that as well. Also include all liquids consumed, as well as any and all snacks that you may have munched on in the last sixty minutes. Do not include any foods that you know, with certainty, did not cause your acid reflux. Your final list of foods should narrow over time as you begin to isolate your trigger foods.

How Much You Consumed

It is important to write down how much you ate with each meal. You can summarize this by using three basic categories: light, moderate or heavy. Light would be a snack, moderate is an appropriately-sized meal, and heavy would indicate that you ate too much.

Activity

Write down a summary of your activities since your last meal. For example, did you eat "on the run," going from appointment to appointment, or were you just relaxing and watching TV? Your activity or non-activity level is important, and should be documented following all GERD episodes. Even being aware of small actions might help you to understand your triggers. Did you take a nap after lunch? Were you exercising? Did you bend over with a full stomach? Ideally, you should write down any physical activity that may have contributed to your reflux episode.

Time

Noting the time of day or night of your last meal, as well as the time of your acid reflux episode, is crucial. This will help to pinpoint the timing of your symptoms following meals, and whether you have daytime or nighttime issues, or both.

Magnitude of Episode and Duration

Rank (using a scale of 1-5) how harsh the episode was. Were you forced to change your plans due to the power of the symptoms? Did you experience moderate discomfort? Was it only a quick burn or did the pain persist for a long period? Determine your own level of magnitude for each rank, with 1 being mild and 5 being harsh.

For this plan you will need some form of recordkeeping capability handy at all times. Smartphones are ideal for jotting down quick information. If you do not have a smartphone, a pocket notebook will also work. We recommend keeping this journal for at least three to four weeks, or until you believe you have identified at least ninety percent of the foods and activities that trigger your reflux episodes.

Visit www.refluxmd.com/gerd-diet-forms to print sample pages for option 1.

Option 2: The Full Journal

As stated previously, this food journaling plan is much more comprehensive in scope and delves deeper into the discovery of triggers and behaviors that may cause symptoms. This plan takes many additional factors into consideration, such as psychology, location, detailed descriptions of symptoms and medications. This is a daily journal that requires more information for each entry, which provides greater analysis.

To start this plan, it is very important to answer two key questions. First, are you currently aware of any foods that are causing your GERD symptoms? Second, if so, why are you eating those items? The first question is typically much easier to answer than the second question, because this behavior is in many cases driven by social factors, emotional issues, situational settings and your personal thoughts (psychological factors). Consider these questions:

- Do you ignore your diet plans when you dine out with friends?

- Do you experience ravenous urges to eat when you feel stress, frustration, boredom, etc.?

- When dining out, do you select foods that are different from those you prepare at home?

- Do you skip certain meals and/or rush through others?

These are just a few of the types of issues you will begin to examine with this wider-ranging food journal.

What to Include in Your Journal

We recommend the following format:

Element	Description
Time?	This is critical, relative to symptom onset.
Food?	Food with a description (fried vs. baked, for example).
Reason?	Hunger, family meal, outside event, mindless eating for no reason
Portion size?	Small, moderate, large.
Pace of meal?	Slow, moderate or rapid.
Emotions?	Frustration, depression, loneliness, boredom, stress, etc.
Where?	Home, work, restaurant, friend's house, etc.
With whom?	Alone, with family, friends, coworkers, clients, etc.
Symptoms?	Nature of symptoms (heartburn, regurgitation, chest pain, etc.), severity (mild, moderate, severe)
Medications?	When, what kind, dosage
Magnitude?	Pain and severity (rank 1-5)
Activity?	Post-meal exercise, post-meal nap, etc.

Visit www.refluxmd.com/gerd-diet-forms to print sample pages for option 2.

How to Use this Journal

You will need to record enough data to be able to draw conclusions about your diet, your behaviors, your emotions, your situations and your symptoms. With this journal, we encourage you to record information about your meals and symptoms for at least one month, and we strongly suggest you take a much longer-term view using this process.

Six Recommendations for Recording Data

1. <u>Record your data as soon as possible.</u> Try to post your data as quickly as possible so you do not forget anything, within ninety minutes of a meal. Your memories may not reflect reality if you wait longer. Maintaining your journal each day will not only help you to gather accurate data, it will also help to reinforce your commitment to the process. If you have a smartphone, set an alarm for typical meal times each day to remind you to record your data.

2. <u>Be honest and accurate.</u> Remember that bad data may result in false conclusions. Recording your emotional state may be the most difficult, but it may also prove to be the most meaningful.

3. <u>Be open with others.</u> Let family, friends and coworkers know what you are doing and what your goals are. Not only will this enable them to understand your actions, but they might also be able to provide additional encouragement and insight.

4. <u>Record your symptoms when they begin.</u> If you wake up at night with GERD symptoms, take a moment to record them and also look at the clock to record the time.

5. <u>Make an initial commitment to recording.</u> Since recording data may at times be difficult and somewhat disruptive, select a distinct time period and make sure you record everything.

6. <u>Start analyzing your data.</u> Start looking for trends any time after seven to ten days.

Interpret the Data in Your Trigger Journal

What can you expect to learn as you interpret the information in your journal?

Here is where you get to play Sherlock Holmes and exercise your acute deductive logic and reasoning skills. This part is just as important as the journal recordkeeping. This is where you have to make sense of the data that will lead to important changes and reduced symptoms.

1. <u>Several trigger foods will begin to surface.</u> For example, chocolate is a trigger food for many, but it is often missed since it is consumed only occasionally, usually in small quantities in the afternoon or evening. If GERD symptoms follow your chocolate consumption, you should realize the relationship over time if you have kept a detailed journal. You may also find out that your favorite steakhouse is not your stomach's favorite. If you track each cup of coffee, you may be surprised to learn that the occasional extra cup creates a problem for you.

2. <u>Certain trends may be apparent.</u> You may notice that Friday nights seem to be more problematic than other nights. Take a look at your Friday activities and determine if there is any change in your behavior: Do you tend to eat out on Friday evenings? Do you drink a bit more wine or other types of alcohol at the end of the work week? Do you eat later on Fridays or recline earlier? With good data and corresponding analysis on your part, these

triggers should become obvious.

3. <u>You may find that your emotions play a role as well.</u> Did that presentation at work create additional stress? When your spouse was on that business trip for ten days, did loneliness result in overeating? Many people find that boredom experienced during the week (or on the weekend) results in "mindless" eating that can often result in GERD symptoms.

4. <u>Other factors may correlate with your GERD symptoms.</u> Did late nights at the office cause you to eat dinner later than usual, triggering nighttime symptoms? Do you experience more symptoms when you eat lunch out with your coworkers? Do you tend to experience symptoms when you get together? When you socialize? On weekends with your friends or neighbors?

5. <u>Master List:</u> Make a separate list of triggers alongside your journal, update it regularly and continue to cross off items as you go. At the end of the journaling process, you should have an excellent idea of the foods and activities that cause your acid reflux. In addition, writing out this list will serve as a good memory exercise. Creating a written list will help to cement these triggers in your memory, making you more aware of them in the future.

Commit to Changing Your Diet to Reduce Your GERD Symptoms
Are You Ready to Make a Change?

It is important to note that we have dedicated the whole of Section IV of this book to overcoming behavior change necessary to successfully achieve GERD relief. Using methods outlined by Dr. Michael Edelstein, a clinical practicing psychologist and published author, we describe a unique and proven approach that goes well beyond the basic methods outlined below.

Eating habits are one of the most challenging aspects of human behavior to change, so make sure you are ready to take on this task before you begin your journal. Based on our communications with RefluxMD members and visitors, everyone seems to fall somewhere on the following spectrum of preparedness:

1. *Change-resistant* – The largest segment of adults. Most desire improved results but are not ready to make the commitment.

2. *Contemplative* – A smaller segment, committed to change that ranges from mild engagement to serious contemplation.

3. *Preparing* – Those who are setting goals and making plans to seek some aspect of behavioral change in the future.

Before you begin this type of program, you will need to be honest about your status. Changing your eating behavior can be difficult. This is a long-term process that should be viewed as a lifelong commitment. In life, things of true value usually do not happen fast or without a great deal of effort. This is especially true for the process of changing eating habits that are typically ingrained in us over a long period of time, often starting in early childhood.

Because everyone is different, almost any food can be a trigger food for someone. Either of these journaling styles should help you to begin to identify the foods that are problematic, and help you to understand when and why you consume certain foods. Eliminating the trigger foods that you have identified from your diet may seem easy, but unless you understand why and when you eat those trigger foods, your long-term behavior may betray you. For example, patterns of eating chocolate and "comfort foods" like cheeseburgers when you are under stress, or consuming alcohol when you are under pressure, need to be recognized and avoided in the future. Gaining this type of knowledge of yourself can be enlightening. With this knowledge you may be more effective in understanding the causes of your GERD symptoms and the behaviors that drive them.

Alcohol and Smoking: Major Causes of Reflux Disease

How much does alcohol consumption contribute to the growth of GERD in the U.S.? According to a July 2012 Gallup survey[28], two thirds of all adults reported they consumed alcohol occasionally. Of these, twenty-two percent indicated that they "drank too much," which was a five percent increase from the year before. Men reported more alcohol consumption, at an average of 6.2 drinks per week, compared to women who reported consuming 2.2 drinks per week. But how does consuming alcohol impact the LES and result in GERD symptoms?

Alcohol consumption is one activity that has been studied and found to have a direct impact on the LES. Many heartburn sufferers report that their symptoms routinely occur after drinking alcohol. In a study by Dr. Kaufman and Dr. Kay titled "Induction of gastroesophageal reflux by alcohol" published in *GUT*, a leading journal in gastroenterology, healthy young adults were given either 180ml of vodka or 180ml of water to determine the impact of alcohol consumption on the LES. A significant difference was found between the two groups, and the researchers concluded that even small quantities of alcohol sometimes triggered GERD symptoms, even in healthy adults. The message is pretty clear: if you want to avoid GERD symptoms, steer clear of obvious triggers like alcoholic beverages.

---

[28] *Saad, Lydia. "Majority in U.S. Drink Alcohol, Averaging Four Drinks a Week." Gallup. 17 Aug 2012.*

The Role of Smoking in GERD Symptoms and Progression

Cigarette smoking has been linked with reducing the function of the LES. Dr. Kahrilas and Dr. Gupta wrote an article published in *GUT* titled "Mechanisms of acid reflux associated with cigarette smoking," which studied smokers and nonsmokers. They concluded that "cigarette smoking probably exacerbates reflux disease by directly provoking acid reflux and perhaps by a long lasting reduction of the lower esophageal sphincter pressure." Although tobacco use in the U.S. has declined over the last twenty years, nineteen percent of all U.S. adults still smoke cigarettes, according to the CDC[29]. Once again, the results of the research are fairly specific: smoking cessation may slow the progression of the disease and may reduce symptoms.

Tips for Changing Your Behavior

Given the current rates of alcohol consumption and tobacco use, it is no surprise that 44%[30] of adults experience GERD symptoms monthly! If we are unable to reduce this level of occurrence in the future, it is possible that GERD will become an epidemic, affecting more adults than any other chronic disease. But what can you do if you want to quit these habits? Here are some tips that can help you get started, and that may improve your chances of success.

Know Your Triggers That Drive the Behavior

Everyone who smokes and/or drinks has triggers that stimulate the urge to partake in these activities. Here are some common triggers that might drive your behavior:

- Emotions such as stress, loneliness, anger, or depression
- Surroundings/setting/location (such as a bar, sporting event, etc.)
- Pre- or post-meal period
- Work breaks
- Quiet time like watching TV or talking on the phone
- Others consuming alcohol or smoking together

Respond to the Urges

It is impossible to avoid all of these potential triggers, so it is important to know how to respond when you begin to sense a craving. Here are some ideas that you can try when the urge hits:

1. **Deep breathing**: Do this multiple times to relax and take your mind off the urge.

2. **Do something else**: chewing gum or drinking water. Others like to read a

[29] *Centers for Disease Control and Prevention. Current Cigarette Smoking Among Adults—United States, 2005–2013.. Morbidity and Mortality Weekly Report 2014;63(47):1108–12 [accessed 2015 Jan 22]*

[30] *P Gorecki, M.D..Gastro-esophageal reflux disease (GERD). Department of Surgery, Nassau University Medical Center.*

magazine or work on a puzzle. Since these urges typically only last for a few moments, find something to distract yourself.

3. **Remind yourself why you are quitting**: The reasons for quitting are a great argument for why you should not give in to the urge!

4. **Phone a friend**: Call someone supportive who wants to help you to quit the behavior.

5. **Exercise**: If you cannot go to the gym or jog around the block, walk up and down the stairs or do sit-ups instead!

6. **Count your savings**: Think about how much money you will save each week, month and year by quitting smoking or drinking.

Nicotine Replacement Therapy for Smoking

Smoking cessation is not simply a behavioral challenge, but a chemical challenge as well. Nicotine can be an addictive chemical and gradual reduction may be helpful to effectively stop smoking. There are several means available to replace nicotine, such as gum, patches, nasal sprays and inhalers. If you use one of these products, you should reduce the dosage over time according to the directions on the package inserts, or consult a qualified healthcare professional.

Join a Program to Help You Quit

You do not have to do this alone. There are many organizations that can assist you to stop smoking or cease the use of alcohol. For example, GlaxoSmithKline offers an online program called Committed Quitters, which is centered around using their nicotine replacement products. The NIH offers a free online program called Smokefree.gov that includes SmokefreeTXT, "a mobile text messaging service designed for adults and young adults across the United States who are trying to quit smoking... created to provide 24/7 encouragement, advice, and tips to help smokers quit smoking and stay quit." There are many programs to assist those seeking to stop the use of alcohol as well. The best known is Alcoholics Anonymous, and there are several others such as SMART Recovery and Rethinking Drinking, a self-help program.

There are many resources available to assist those committed to changing a habit or a lifestyle. We recommend that you explore the alternatives by doing an Internet search to identify a program that makes sense to you.

Get Started Today by Scheduling a Visit With Your Physician

Your doctor can add substantial value to your efforts and will have access to resources that can help you to succeed. Withdrawal from either smoking or alcohol use can put stress on your body, so your doctor should be part of your team to design an effective program.

Take Your Time, Build Your Team, Design Your Plan and Get Started

We realize that this may be the most difficult and the most challenging lifestyle change for you to make over the long run. **But it can be done.** This is not a decision that should be taken lightly or jumped into quickly. Rather, take your time to design a program that you think will work for you. Work with your physician, family, friends and coworkers to provide additional advice and support. Remember, the harder the challenge, the more valuable the reward. Good luck!

Section III
A Step-By-Step Approach

Section III: Overview

"This is where theory meets reality. We will explain our step-by-step approach to managing your diet in a way that is easy to implement."

Now that you have a better understanding of the importance of managing your diet to reduce your GERD symptoms, it is time to get to work on building your diet plan! This is where theory meets reality. In the following chapters we will explain our step-by-step approach to managing your diet in a way that is easy to implement. **For the next step, please print MY PERSONAL PLAN from http://www.refluxmd.com/gerd-diet-forms, so you can record your assessment and goals.**

Chapter 16 – Preliminary Assessment

This chapter is designed to help you to make an honest assessment of where you stand today, creating a clear picture of your personal baseline that will allow you to measure your success over time. We explain how to gather key information that you should record prior to starting any diet program.

Chapter 17 – Setting Goals

This chapter highlights the importance of setting goals to achieve long-term success. We assist you in establishing several goals, including weight loss and symptom reduction, and setting realistic timeframes to achieve them. Each goal will be measurable, for the purpose of tracking success.

Chapter 18 – Tracking

Being able to measure your goals is important not only for tracking your progress, but for providing psychological encouragement as well. In this chapter we describe weekly tracking of key data and compare it to established weekly goals.

Chapter 19 – Good Eating Habits

In this chapter we discuss eating habits and meal-planning strategies for success.

Chapter 20 – Reading Food Labels

Here we provide information on food labels: how to read them and use them as a guide.

Chapter 21 – Keep Stress Low

Since any lifestyle change can bring on stress, this chapter offers strategies for managing that stress, so it does not derail your plan.

Chapter 16
Preliminary Assessment

Find Your Current Body Mass Index (BMI)

Since assessment of BMI is vital for measuring progress, we repeat the table and some of the discussion found in Section II here. BMI is a measurement that uses weight and height to assess body weight. BMI is often used as a tool to determine whether you are at a healthy weight or not. It is a quick and easy way to determine where you are today, and can help you to pick a healthier target weight to achieve. To determine your BMI, find your approximate height on the vertical axis and your weight within the chart below to determine your BMI. For example, a 6'2" person who 218 pounds has a BMI of 28.

BMI Chart

BMI	21	22	23	24	25	26	27	28	29	30	31
4'10"	100	105	110	115	119	124	129	134	138	143	148
4'11"	104	109	114	119	124	128	133	138	143	148	153
5'0"	107	112	118	123	128	133	138	143	148	153	158
5'1"	111	116	122	127	132	137	143	148	153	158	164
5'2"	115	120	126	131	136	142	147	153	158	164	169
5'3"	118	124	130	135	141	146	152	158	163	169	175
5'4"	122	128	134	140	145	151	157	163	169	174	180
5'5"	126	132	138	144	150	156	162	168	174	180	186
5'6"	130	136	142	148	155	161	167	173	179	186	192
5'7"	134	140	146	153	159	166	172	178	185	191	198
5'8"	138	144	151	158	164	171	177	184	190	197	203
5'9"	142	149	155	162	169	176	182	189	196	203	209
5'10"	146	153	160	167	174	181	188	195	202	209	216
5'11"	150	157	165	172	179	186	193	200	208	215	222
6'0"	154	162	169	177	184	191	199	206	213	221	228
6'1"	159	166	174	182	189	197	204	212	219	227	235
6'2"	163	171	179	186	194	202	210	218	225	233	241
6'3"	168	176	184	192	200	208	216	224	232	240	248

Normal weight relative to height: BMI of 18.5 to 24.9
Overweight relative to height: BMI of 25.0 to 29.9
Obese relative to height: BMI of 30 or higher
For a more accurate BMI calculation, please visit the NIH website to access their BMI calculator.

Once you have determined your BMI, be sure to record it on the form titled MY PERSONAL PLAN in the box for "Starting BMI." Also record your current weight in the box for "Starting Body Weight."

MY PERSONAL PLAN is available at http://www.refluxmd.com/gerd-diet-forms.

Measure Your Current Waist Circumference

In Section II we talked about how excessive belly fat can cause symptoms of acid reflux, but did you know that excess belly fat also increases your risk for heart disease and cancer? As a result, reducing your waist circumference is an important goal for your overall health. To find this measurement, simply wrap a flexible tape measure (or a belt or piece of string, if you do not have one) around your midsection, even with or just above your belly button. Take this measurement before you have consumed any food for the day, relaxing your stomach muscles. Once you have that measurement, in inches and centimeters, enter that into your form titled MY PERSONAL PLAN in the box for "Starting Waist Circumference."

Determine Your Current Calorie Consumption

Everyone who suffers from reflux disease does not necessarily need to cut calories out of his/her diet, but understanding the calories in the foods you eat can help you to make healthier choices and manage your weight over time, whether you need to lose weight or are already at a healthy weight and want to maintain it.

To put our diet plan into action, you will need to determine your daily calorie needs. This varies depending on your age, sex, current height and weight, and activity level. The following chart provides a rough estimate of the number of calories you will need each day. A variety of additional tools are available online to help you calculate this number, such as the Mayo Clinic's Calorie Calculator.

Using the BMI example that we started with, the daily calorie requirement for a sixty-year-old male who is 6'2" tall and weighs 218 pounds, with a "somewhat active" lifestyle (which includes light or moderate activity about two to three times a week), is 2,600 calories. As you can see from the following table, activity levels have a significant impact on daily calorie requirements.

As you'll, calorie requirements can change significantly based upon activity level as well as your current weight. Consequently, if your activity level changes, it is important to re-compute your daily calorie requirement. We recommend that you re-compute this requirement monthly, as your weight begins to change.

Again, the calorie calculator estimates the number of calories you will need every day in order to maintain your current weight. This also serves as a good way to estimate approximately how many calories per day you are currently consuming if your weight has been reasonably steady for the last several weeks. Just remember, this number should not become your goal unless you are happy with your current weight. If your goal is to lose weight, then you will need to gradually reduce the number of calories you eat on a daily basis. Consider this number to be your starting point.

Calorie Requirements to Maintain Weight
for a 6'2" Sixty-Year-Old Male, Based on Activity

Activity Level	Calorie Requirement
Inactive - none or limited daily activity	2,350
Somewhat Active - light or moderate activity 2 or 3 times weekly	2,600
Active - 30 minutes of moderate activity most days OR vigorous activity at least 3 days a week	2,850
Very Active - Significant amount of moderate or vigorous activity daily	3,300

Once you have determined your calorie requirements, enter that number into your form titled MY PERSONAL PLAN in the box for "Starting Calorie Consumption."

Log Your Starting GERD Symptoms

The ultimate goal of this diet plan is to help you to manage your GERD symptoms. Symptoms have two primary elements: severity and frequency. RefluxMD has developed a chart to determine your starting symptom level, which can range from Grade 1 (mild and infrequent) to Grade 7 (frequent and severe). The following guidelines will assist you in determining your symptom grade level throughout your program.

Severity Levels (SL)

Severity	Description
MILD	Awareness of symptoms but easily tolerated.
MODERATE	Discomforting. sufficient to cause interference with normal daily activities, including sleep.
SEVERE	Incapacitating. unable to perform normal daily activities, including sleep.

Frequency Levels (FL)

Frequency	Description
Infrequent	Symptoms 1 day during the past week.
Occasional	Symptoms 2 to 4 days during the past week.
Frequent	Symptoms more than 4 days during the past week.

RefluxMD Symptom Grade Level
Combined Frequency and Severity Levels

	FL - Infrequent	FL - Occasional	FL - Frequent
SL - FREQUENT	Grade 5	Grade 7	Grade 9
SL - MODERATE	Grade 3	Grade 6	Grade 8
SL - MILD	Grade 1	Grade 2	Grade 4

Instructions on the use of this chart

Based on the definitions in the Severity Level chart above, decide the Severity Level that best describes the overall severity of your GERD symptoms (Frequent, Moderate or Mild). Once you have this decided, use the definitions in the Frequency Level chart to decide which Frequency Level best describes the frequency of your GERD episodes (Infrequent, Occasional or Frequent). Now find the column for each and find the cell where each of your two columns meet - and that is your Grade Level. For example, if I have a Severity Level of Moderate and a Frequency Level of Occasional, my Symptom Grade Level is Grade 6.

Your goal should be to completely eliminate all future acid reflux symptoms. Thus, we hope your goal will be to reach Grade 0, with zero symptoms of acid reflux. Using the RefluxMD Symptom Grade Level Chart above, please consider your symptom frequency and severity over the past several weeks and select your Grade Level. Enter this Grade Level into your form titled MY PERSONAL PLAN in the box for "Starting Symptom Grade Level," and place a 0 in the box under "Target Symptom Grade Level." If you do not feel achieving zero symptoms is a reasonable goal, enter a Grade Level that would satisfy you. As you use this chart every week, only consider your symptoms from the previous week.

Identify Your Trigger Foods

In Chapter 4 of Section II, we described how to keep a food journal. We provided two options, depending on how you want to approach tracking your diet and your GERD symptoms. Choose whichever journal works best for you.

If you are not yet aware of your trigger foods, it should take you two weeks to a month to track your diet and identify what triggers your symptoms. However, continuing to track the frequency and magnitude of your GERD symptoms and the medications you take is a good practice, at least during your weight loss period if not indefinitely. This will help you to measure your progress and work with your doctor to tweak your treatment plan, should your condition change.

When you keep your journal, be sure to track both the frequency and the severity of your symptoms. Both categories are important to record. For example, you may find that your symptoms have not changed in frequency at the onset of your new diet, but their magnitude has changed. At this early stage, a reduction of symptoms indicates progress. If you did not record the magnitude of your symptoms, your analysis would fail to show this progress.

On the form titled MY PERSONAL PLAN we have listed KNOWN TRIGGER FOODS. For those that trigger your symptoms, place an "X" in the corresponding box. If you have any other trigger foods or beverages, list those on the form as well.

Congratulations!
You have established a baseline or starting point! Now we need to identify your goals and establish a plan to achieve them.

Chapter 17
Setting Goals

This is not a "cold turkey" approach, nor a plan that looks for immediate results, but rather one that focuses on consistency with slow and steady progress.

In this section you will learn to establish goals based on the data you have collected, as outlined in the previous chapter. Ideally, you will set specific measurable goals in each category, as well as a reasonable timeframe for accomplishing your goals. As mentioned previously, our approach encourages you to work towards your goals at a manageable and gradual pace. This is not a "cold turkey" approach, nor a plan that looks for immediate results, but rather one that focuses on consistency with slow and steady progress. Using this mentality, your plan will aim for regular "base hits" rather than a few "home runs" to win the game.

A Note About Exercise

Staying active is an important part of a healthy lifestyle. As mentioned earlier, calorie consumption tracked to maintain or reduce weight is dependent upon activity levels. While our plan does not specify how or when you should exercise, you will need to consider your activity level when setting your goals because it can impact the number of calories you will need each day. If you want to reduce your BMI, activities that raise your heart rate can help you to burn more calories. If your goal is to reduce your waistline, then get started with cardio exercises to burn calories. We also encourage strengthening your core muscles as a key to improved overall health.

The first step is to see your doctor to get approval to increase your physical activity. Then, establish an activity program that will help you to achieve your desired results. There are many websites, apps and books available to help you get started. You might consider working with a personal trainer to create a fitness plan designed specifically for you. Remember, activity level has an impact on your new targeted calorie consumption:

Somewhat active (S)
Light or moderate activity 2 or 3 times weekly

Active (A)
Half hour of moderate activity most days or vigorous activity at least 3 days weekly

Very Active (V)
Significant amount of moderate or vigorous activity daily

Based on your activity level over the past several weeks, enter an S, A or V into your form titled MY PERSONAL PLAN in the box for "Starting Activity Level," and place another letter in the box under "Target Activity Level" to represent the new activity level that you hope to incorporate in your new diet and lifestyle plan.

BMI and Weight Goals

In Chapter 16, we used the BMI chart (reproduced below) to determine your current BMI. Now we use the same chart to determine your target weight goal, based on BMI. Once this is established, you will determine your goal for daily calorie consumption.

As discussed earlier, BMI is a simple tool used to measure obesity on the following scale:
Normal weight: BMI of 18.5 to 24.9
Overweight: BMI of 25.0 to 29.9
Obese: BMI of 30 or higher

Your goal should be to reduce your BMI to a number within the normal weight range. For example, if your current BMI is 27, a good goal might be to reduce that to 24. Once you have determined your BMI goal, enter it into your form titled MY PERSONAL PLAN in the box titled "Target BMI".

Now, let us go back to that BMI chart to determine your target weight based upon that BMI goal. Locate your height on the vertical axis on the left side of the chart. Then, locate your target BMI goal that you just established on the horizontal axis at the top line of the chart. Where the BMI goal column and your height column intersect on the graph, you will find your target weight goal.

BMI Chart

BMI	21	22	23	24	25	26	27	28	29	30	31
4'10"	100	105	110	115	119	124	129	134	138	143	148
4'11"	104	109	114	119	124	128	133	138	143	148	153
5'0"	107	112	118	123	128	133	138	143	148	153	158
5'1"	111	116	122	127	132	137	143	148	153	158	164
5'2"	115	120	126	131	136	142	147	153	158	164	169
5'3"	118	124	130	135	141	146	152	158	163	169	175
5'4"	122	128	134	140	145	151	157	163	169	174	180
5'5"	126	132	138	144	150	156	162	168	174	180	186
5'6"	130	136	142	148	155	161	167	173	179	186	192
5'7"	134	140	146	153	159	166	172	178	185	191	198

5'8"	138	144	151	158	164	171	177	184	190	197	203
5'9"	142	149	155	162	169	176	182	189	196	203	209
5'10"	146	153	160	167	174	181	188	195	202	209	216
5'11"	150	157	165	172	179	186	193	200	208	215	222
6'0"	154	162	169	177	184	191	199	206	213	221	228
6'1"	159	166	174	182	189	197	204	212	219	227	235
6'2"	163	171	179	186	194	202	210	218	225	233	241
6'3"	168	176	184	192	200	208	216	224	232	240	248

For a more accurate BMI calculation, please visit the NIH website to access their BMI calculator.

Using the same example we used earlier (a sixty-year-old male, 6'2" tall, who would like to achieve a BMI of 24), read across from the height of 6'2" and then read down from a BMI of 24. The number found here those two columns intersect is his target weight, or 186 pounds.

Once you have determined your own target weight using your target BMI and your height, please enter that weight into your form titled MY PERSONAL PLAN in the box for "Target Body Weight".

Targeted Weight Loss in Pounds

Once you have determined your target weight, figure out how many pounds you need to lose to achieve that goal. This computation is simple. Just subtract your target weight from your current weight to find out how many pounds you need to lose. For some people, that number will be zero if they are already at their target or healthy weight. Determine your total weight loss goal and on MY PERSONAL PLAN, compute that number in the box "Total Weight Loss".

Calories

Now that you have set your BMI and weight goals, you can figure out how many calories per day you should eat to achieve that goal. Your daily goal is based upon how quickly you want to lose weight. As a general rule, most physicians and dieticians recommend losing weight at a rate of no more than one to two pounds each week. Be realistic about how much weight you will lose weekly. Losing too much too quickly can result in muscle loss rather than fat loss, which is not what we are trying to accomplish. Losing just half a pound each week will require less dietary disruption and may result in less hunger pains and an easier adjustment than may be required in order to lose two pounds each week. With that said, the required dieting timeframe is going to be four times longer at a weight loss rate of half a pound per week versus two pounds per week to achieve the same results. Only you can determine what is best for you. Remember, you have to create a "calorie deficit" to lose weight, which means that you must burn more calories than you consume. One pound of lost weight equals approximately 3,500 more calories burned each week than calories consumed each week. Reducing calorie consumption by 500 calories each day from your current diet should result in one pound of weight loss per a week (500 calories x 7 = 3,500 calories). By reducing calorie consumption by 1,000 calories each day, the projected weight loss would double to two pounds lost that week. However, as a guideline, we suggest that women should consume a minimum of 1,200 calories each day, and men should go no lower than 1,500 calories daily.

Let us return to the example of our 6'2" 218-pound sixty-year-old male. With an activity level of "somewhat active," calorie consumption to maintain his current weight was estimated to be 2,600 calories. Assuming weight loss targets between half a pound and two pounds each week, you can begin to understand the corresponding challenges involved when aiming to lose weight faster:

Targeted weekly weight loss	Required calorie reduction	% of current 2,600 calorie consumption
0.5 Pounds	250 Daily	9.6%
1.0 Pounds	500 Daily	19.2%
1.5 Pounds	750 Daily	28.8%
2.0 Pounds	1,000 Daily	38.5%

This chart highlights the challenge of adopting a more aggressive weight loss rate. For this sixty-year-old to lose 1.5 pounds each week, he would have to reduce his consumption by almost thirty percent, which may prove to be too difficult. As you can see, it may be even more difficult to achieve the 2.0 pounds per week goal. However, losing between 0.5 pounds and 1.0 pounds weekly may be more manageable because this requires eating only ten to twenty percent fewer calories each week.

There is one additional factor to consider if you plan to increase your daily activity level. Since exercise can also burn calories that are counted towards your goal, you might also consider factoring this into the equation as well. A free calorie burning calculator tool is available at Health Status, which may be useful in this analysis.

Staying with our sixty-year-old male, let us assume that he is adding a daily walk of thirty minutes at about three miles per hour to his activity schedule. Using the Health Status calculator, this would result in approximately 215 more calories burned daily.

Assuming our sixty-year-old plans to lose 1.5 pounds per week, he must burn 750 calories more than he consumes. However, 215 of that total will be achieved through exercise. His new calorie reduction target is noted below:

Targeted weekly weight loss:	1.5 pounds
Daily calorie reduction:	750
Calorie burn – walking:	215
Reduced calories – diet:	535
% of current diet:	20.6%

By adding exercise or other activities to his diet program, he can maximize his weight loss with less impact on this diet.

We encourage you to target a daily calorie reduction, from reduced consumption and increased activity, of between 300 and 800 calories less than your current daily consumption/burn rate. We want to stress again that this is a personal decision. Use the calorie calculation to determine your weekly calorie reduction on MY PERSONAL PLAN, and compute the "Reduced Calories From Diet".

Waist Circumference Goals

In general, men with a waist circumference of more than 40 inches, and non-pregnant women with a waist circumference greater than 35 inches, may be at a higher risk of developing obesity-related illnesses. For most adults, your target waist circumference may be found with a simple calculation. As a general rule, your ideal waist measurement should be less than half your height. For example, our sixty-year-old male is 6'2" or 74 inches tall. He should have a waist circumference of 37 inches or less. We have created the following chart so you can easily determine your waistline goal. Locate your height and then note the corresponding waist circumference goal. If your height is not listed in the table, simply divide your height (in inches) by two.

Keep in mind that this number only serves as a guideline. Some people have larger or smaller frames than others. Use this figure as a starting point and determine YOUR goal based on your judgment and/or in conjunction with your doctor. Once you have determined your ideal waist size, please enter it into your form titled MY PERSONAL PLAN in the box for "Target Waist Circumference".

Targeted Waist Circumference Based on Height and Weight (in Inches)

Height	Inches	Targeted Circumference
5' 0"	60	30.0
5' 1"	61	30.5
5' 2"	62	31.0
5' 3"	63	31.5
5' 4"	64	32.0
5' 5"	65	32.5
5' 6"	66	33.0
5' 7"	67	33.5
5' 8"	68	34.0
5' 9"	69	34.5
5' 10"	70	35.0
5' 11"	71	35.5
6' 0"	72	36.0
6' 1"	73	36.5
6' 2"	74	37.0
6' 3"	75	37.5

Designing the Week-by-week Plan

Before we start building your week-by-week plan, it is important to note that weight loss is not going to be consistent every week. Your body is complicated with lots of things going on all the time, so you will experience weeks where you lose more pounds than you expected, and weeks where you remain the same weight despite your best efforts. Keep your weekly (and daily) goals in perspective. You will succeed over the long term, but maybe not in a straight line.

To determine how many weeks you will need to lose weight to achieve your goal, simply divide the total weight loss goal by the targeted weekly weight loss. The result will determine how many weeks are required to achieve your total weight loss goal. Life does not always allow us to stay on our diet programs week after week. Vacations, celebrations, weddings, etc. can result in a lost week. Plan for one "setback" week every two months (or approximately every eight or nine weeks).

Using the example of our sixty-year-old male, we will determine how many weeks of weight loss are required to go from his current weight of 218 down to 186 pounds.

Current weight	218 pounds
Less target weight	186 pounds
= Total weight loss	32 pounds
Divided by targeted weekly weight loss	1.5 pounds per week
= "Theoretical" # of weeks	21 weeks (or approx. 5 months)
Lost weeks (1 per every 2 months)	3 weeks (rounded up from 2.5)
= Total weeks to lose all weight	24 weeks (rounded up from 23.7)

With a 24-week program and a goal of losing 1.5 pounds per week (with almost three lost weeks), here is our weekly plan for targeted weight goals:

Target Weight at the End of Each Week

Week	1	2	3	4	5	6	7	8
Weight Goal	216.5	215.0	213.5	212.0	210.5	209.0	207.5	206.0
Weight Lost (Goal)	1.5	3.0	4.5	6.0	7.5	9.0	10.5	12.0
Actual Weight								
Actual Total Lost								
Actual Waist Size								

Week	9	10	11	12	13	14	15	16
Weight Goal	206.0	204.5	203.0	201.5	200.0	198.5	197.0	195.5
Weight Lost (Goal)	12.0	13.5	15.0	16.5	18.0	19.5	21.0	22.5
Actual Weight								
Actual Total Lost								
Actual Waist Size								

Week	17	18	19	20	21	22	23	24
Weight Goal	194.0	194.0	192.5	191.0	189.5	188.0	186.5	186.0
Weight Lost (Goal)	24.0	24.0	25.5	27.0	28.7	30.0	31.5	32.0
Actual Weight								
Actual Total Lost								

If you want to track your weight loss progress weekly, complete the Weekly Diet Plan Chart available at http://www.refluxmd.com/gerd-diet-forms.

Chapter 18
Tracking

"Tracking will help you to assess your progress and keep you motivated as you work toward your goals."

Taking the time to track your progress is essential to achieving your goals. Tracking will help you to assess your progress and keep you motivated as you work toward your goals. By keeping daily records, your commitment will be strengthened and your enthusiasm will increase.

BMI and Weight

Tracking your BMI and weight is simple and requires only a scale. Just before bed at the end of every week, weigh yourself and record it on your RefluxMD Weekly Weight Plan Chart. Keep in mind that your weight may fluctuate three to five pounds throughout the day/week, so try to weigh yourself at the same time each week using the same scale for the most accurate comparison from week to week. Because of that fluctuation, you may not notice much of a change for the first few weeks. Hang in there. If you stick with the program, you WILL see results and you will start to see a downward trend in your weight.

Waistline

Changes in your waistline will happen slowly because a considerable amount of weight loss is required before it may be noticeable. For the average female to lose one inch of waistline she would have to lose five to seven pounds, and the average man would have to lose eight to ten pounds. Because of that, we suggest you only measure your waist once every four weeks using the same method that was used the first time you measured your waistline, and record that number in your Weekly Weight Plan Chart. Patience is a virtue here, but when you do see progress it will feel very rewarding.

Calories

Not so excited about counting calories? Do not worry! It does not have to be cumbersome. There are some great methods to help you keep track of what you are eating every day.

The simplest method is to plan out your meals ahead of time. By planning your meals, you can calculate how many calories you will be eating. If you stick to your plan, you will know how many you consumed every day or week. To help you get started, we have created twenty-one daily meal plans with eighty different recipes that include various breakfasts, lunches, dinners and snacks. Each meal plan includes a detailed nutritional breakdown, so you will know exactly what you are getting with each meal. Over time you will become more comfortable with these daily meal plans and may begin to modify them and/or build them yourself.

If you are not much of a planner or you prefer to do your own thing, counting your calories each day may be accomplished as an easy extension of your food journal. Since you are already recording your meals, you will just need to figure out how many calories are in each food or beverage you consume. There are a variety of free tools available online today that can help you here. These apps and websites provide massive amounts of data to help you look up the nutritional information for your favorite foods (including items from your favorite restaurants) and keep a running tally of your daily intake. Two of our favorites are the MyPlate calorie counter on livestrong.com and the My Fitness Pal app for your smartphone. Both require you to register but are free to use.

Whichever method you prefer, this record keeping process will greatly assist you in losing weight and achieving your health goals.

Symptom Tracking

You should continue tracking your symptoms in your food journal. Each week, you should record your Symptom Stage based on frequency and severity over the past seven days. Over time, this number should significantly decrease.

One final note on tracking: Review your results without emotions; do not be annoyed or take offense if they are not what you were hoping to see. Do not get discouraged if your results do not show immediate progress or if they reverse or even increase for a week or two. With diligence, effort and time, you will eventually achieve your desired results.

Chapter 19
Good Eating Habits

"Small changes can help to get you headed in the right direction! Keep in mind, the first week of a new "habit" is the hardest, but if you stick with it, your new habit will eventually become a natural part of your routine."

In this chapter, we explore the habits that can help you make long-term, healthy changes to your diet. Long-term success with any diet program requires a hard look at your current eating habits, so that you can come up with a plan to overcome the bad ones (we all have them) and create new healthier ones. All of the habits outlined here may not fit into your lifestyle, but they should give you some ideas about how you can tweak your habits to improve your health. Feel free to customize them to work for you. For example, we suggest bringing your lunch to work. If this seems unreasonable, set a goal to bring your lunch three days a week to start. Small changes can help to get you headed in the right direction! Keep in mind the first week of a new "habit" is the hardest, but if you stick with it, your new habit will eventually become a natural part of your routine.

Plan Your Meals

Meal planning can take a little time up front, but it can actually save time overall and make day-to-day life much simpler. Planning what you will eat ahead of time can help you stick to your goals, and can eliminate the daily stress associated with the frequent question, "what am I going to eat?" It can also guide your choices at the grocery store, all of which means you will be less likely to make a bad choice when you are tired and/or hungry. Spend a little time planning your meals days (or even weeks!) ahead of time. Then, all you have to do is follow your plan and you will be on your way to meeting your goals and progressing toward optimal health.

In this book we have included twenty-one daily meal plans and eighty different acid reflux-friendly recipes to help you get started. Each recipe includes detailed nutritional information, to make sure you know exactly what you are eating. You can choose to follow our meal plans exactly or adapt them to suit your needs. The key is to create a meal plan that is well-balanced and easy for you to follow. Also, be sure to keep a few quick, easy and healthy favorites (like an omelet loaded with veggies, a quick stir-fry, etc.) in your back pocket for days when your plan is derailed (i.e. you are late coming home from the office, you ran out of a key ingredient or you just do not feel like eating what you had planned).

Cook at Home

People eat out for a variety of reasons – it is social, quick and easy to grab something on a busy day. Also, many adults simply do not like to cook. However, the downside to eating out is that restaurant meals are often loaded with sugar, fat and sodium, and the portion sizes can be unusually large. If you eat out frequently, it will be more difficult for you to stick with your healthy eating plan and your weight loss efforts may suffer, not to mention your acid reflux. As a result, we strongly encourage you to cook at home as much as possible. By cooking your own meals, you have complete control over what you eat, and you will be more likely to pick healthy ingredients and avoid unhealthy foods.

When you do choose to eat out, use caution and try not to overdo it. Take a look at the menu beforehand to identify a few healthier choices on the menu, so you will be less likely to give in to temptation when you sit down at the table. Many restaurants are now required to offer nutritional information on their menus, so it is easier to identify choices that fit into your diet plan. If your portion is huge, remember this – you do not have to eat it all. Consider wrapping up half for lunch the next day or opting for a small portion instead.

Include Snacks in Your Plan

Healthy snacks are an important part of your diet plan because they can help to keep you feeling satisfied throughout the day, and you will not be tempted to overindulge at your next meal. Since hunger can be overwhelming and lead to impulsive eating, snacks can help to manage your appetite and keep you on track. As with your meals, planning your snacks will ensure that you have healthy choices on hand and are not tempted by the vending machine or corner store when hunger strikes. Just be sure to keep snacks at a reasonable size so that they do not inadvertently turn into full meals. Here are several ideas to get you started:

- *Cottage Cheese and Apples:* Simply core a golden delicious or red apple, cut it into small slices, and add ½ cup of low-fat cottage cheese.

- *Edamame:* Steam or boil ½ cup of shelled baby soybeans and add a touch of salt to taste.

- *Banana:* The most transportable snack of all. It even comes in its own protective cover.

- *Baby Carrots and Hummus:* Baby carrots are easy to find and require no preparation. 1½ cups is an appropriately-sized portion. To add some spice and protein to the snack, serve with 2 Tbsp. of hummus.

- *Hard-boiled Egg with Toast:* Easy to prepare ahead of time. When you are ready to eat, just slice it up and place the slices on a toasted piece of whole wheat bread.

- *Nonfat Greek Yogurt:* Find a plain or flavored Greek yogurt and snack on ½ cup. Add some fruit for a little kick to the taste buds and added fiber.

- *Almonds:* Snack on 8 to 10 plain or lightly salted almonds.

- *Grapes:* Typically 25 to 30 grapes in a cup, and they make a refreshing and tasty snack.

- *Celery with Peanut butter:* Quick, easy and fun to eat!

- *Cheese and Crackers:* Try 4 to 6 whole grain crackers with low fat or fat-free cheese.

- *Granola with Fruit:* 1 cup of granola with a few strawberries or blueberries.

- *Popcorn:* Cups of popcorn is an appropriately-sized serving, plain, lightly salted or topped with your favorite spices.

- *Melba Toast Crackers:* 4 or 5 crackers, either rye or pumpernickel.

- *Instant Pudding:* Use fat-free and sugar-free pudding mix and make with nonfat milk.

- *Bagel and Peanut butter:* Spread peanut butter on ½ a whole wheat bagel.

- *Avocado:* Half of an avocado makes a high fiber snack that is rich in omega-3 fats.

- *Fresh Vegetables:* 1 cup of your favorite veggie such as cucumbers, mushrooms, celery or broccoli.

- *Grape Nuts and Yogurt:* ⅓ cup of Grape Nuts with 4 oz of nonfat yogurt.

- *Pistachios:* Eat 20 to 25. Time spent removing the shells will slow down your appetite!

- *Sunflower Seeds:* 1 cup. Like pistachios, removing the shells will slow you down!

Bring Your Lunch

Extend your meal planning to include your lunch. By preparing and bringing a lunch to work, you can control exactly what and how much you eat. As discussed earlier, eating out frequently can quickly sabotage your efforts. While there is nothing wrong with the occasional lunch out with your coworkers, you will see better results if you make bringing a healthy lunch with you to work a habit.

Reduce Your Portion Sizes

As mentioned earlier, managing portion size is an essential part of combating GERD. Overfilling your stomach can lead to painful symptoms, so reducing your portion sizes can dramatically impact how you feel. Our meal plans and recipes include proper portion sizes, and if you stick with the recommended portions, no further adjustments are necessary. If you eat out or decide to try a new recipe, be mindful of how much food you put on your plate and eat slowly. It takes about twenty minutes for your brain to recognize that your stomach is full, so eating more slowly gives your brain a chance to catch up with your stomach. Another simple idea is to set your fork down on your plate between each bite. Take it slow, make eye contact with your meal partners, enjoy their company, and engage in conversation before you take the next bite.

Chapter 20
Reading Food Labels

Understanding food labels, how to read them, and how to use the information provided, will help you to make healthier decisions when navigating the grocery store aisles. Once you understand how to read and interpret these labels, you may be surprised at how much fat, sodium, sugar and cholesterol is in many of your favorite foods. These labels are ideal for comparison-shopping, for those seeking the healthiest selections. This data can help to further your commitment to staying on track and reinforce the selection of healthier options that will help you find relief from reflux. Beware of health claims on product packaging. By reading the label, you may be surprised to discover that the brand claiming "LOW SODIUM" might not be the best option for you. For more information on food labels, visit the FDA website.

Most packaged foods are required to have a Nutrition Facts label that looks something like this:

Nutrition Facts

Serving Size 1/2 cup (115g)
Servings Per Container About 4

Amount Per Serving

Calories 250	Calories from Fat 130

	% Daily Value*
Total Fat 14g	**22%**
Saturated Fat 9g	**45%**
Cholesterol 55mg	**18%**
Sodium 75mg	**3%**
Total Carbohydrate 26g	**9%**
Dietary Fiber 0g	**0%**
Sugars 26g	
Protein 4g	

Vitamin A 10%	Vitamin C 0%
Calcium 10%	Iron 0%

* Percent Daily Values are based on a 2,000 calorie diet.

Let us discuss each item and explore how you can use it in your food selections.

Serving Size

The first line on the Nutrition Facts label indicates the recommended serving size. Pay attention to this number because it is the key to interpreting the rest of the label. The nutritional information that follows is based upon this serving size. For example, if you are reading a Nutrition Facts label on a package of sliced cheese, the serving size may be "2 slices". This tells you that the nutritional values that follow are based on a two-slice serving – not the entire package. If the label states that there are 10 grams of fat per serving, then you will know that there are 10 grams of fat in only two slices of cheese.

The next item in this section tells you how many servings there are per container. This number is useful because it can help you to determine how much of any nutrient is in the package as a whole. For example, assume you are looking at a can of green beans that you and another person will share for dinner. The label indicates 4 servings, and each serving has 300 mg of sodium. You now know that the whole can has 1200 mg of sodium (4 x 300 mg) and that each of you will consume 600 mg of sodium (either 2 x 300 mg or 1,200/2). Knowing the amount of servings per container can also help you to estimate the size of a serving. You might not know how much three ounces is, but if you know that there are four servings in a 12-ounce package, then you will know that a quarter of the package (which is easier to estimate) is roughly 3 ounces.

Calories

The next line indicates the number of calories per serving. Next to the calories you will find "calories from fat," which indicates how many of the total calories are from fat. For example, if a serving of an item has two hundred calories and one hundred of those calories are from fat, then you may quickly determine that this item is high in fat because it makes up half of the calories. Ultimately, these numbers may help you to track your calories and can help you to make smart shopping decisions. According to the Mayo Clinic[31], ideally twenty to thirty-five percent of your daily calories should come from fat.

If your diet plan calls for 2,000 calories daily, the total calories from fat should be between 400 calories (2,000 x 0.20) and 750 calories (2,000 x 0.35). If you prefer to track fat in grams, just remember that there are 9 calories per gram of fat. In the above example, the daily total calories from fat should be between 44 grams (400/9) and 50 grams (750/9). This range may seem somewhat conservative since the U.S. Food and Drug Administration (FDA) has set the daily reference value for adults who consume 2,000 calories daily at 65 grams. Keep in mind that there are different types of fat. The goal is to consume the majority of fat from a healthier fat source (unsaturated fats) and the least amount possible from unhealthy fat sources (saturated and trans fats) Because fat, whether healthy or unhealthy, contains 9 calories per gram, remember that less is more.

[31] *Mayo Clinic. "Nutrition and Healthy Eating." 7 Aug 2014*

% Daily Value

In the United States, the FDA has created guidelines for the amount of each micronutrient and most macronutrients that are necessary to ensure that your nutritional needs are met. These recommendations are reflected in the % Daily Value section of the Nutrition Facts label. The % Daily Value figure indicates the percentage of the total recommended amount of that nutrient provided by one serving of the food item, based on a 2,000-calorie diet. For example, if a label indicates 14% sodium, that means one serving of that product provides fourteen percent of your recommended daily allowance for sodium. According to the Mayo Clinic[32], it is suggested that a 5% Daily Value is considered low and a 20% Daily Value is considered high for any specific food. The Mayo Clinic also suggests selecting foods that have high % of Daily Values for vitamins, minerals and fiber, but limit foods with high % Daily Values for fat, cholesterol and sodium.

One last note on the % Daily Value: The numbers on the top section of the label are based on a 2,000-calorie diet. A footnote at the bottom of the label will tell you what values are used according to a 2,000 and/or a 2,500-calorie diet. If your daily calorie goal is lower than the referenced value, your % Daily Value will be less, and the opposite if your daily goal is higher. These numbers can help you make quick "ballpark" estimates about what you are eating, but you many not want to focus too heavily on the exact numbers.

Nutrients to Limit

As was just mentioned, it is important to differentiate between fat, cholesterol, sodium, carbohydrates (including sugar and fiber) and protein. These nutrients are all necessary components of your diet, but the top three – fat, cholesterol, and sodium – are generally considered nutrients that should be limited. Remember that these numbers are based on a single serving rather than the whole package.

You will notice that the fat count includes the total amount of fat, as well as how much saturated fat and trans fat the product contains. The American Heart Association (AHA) recommends[33] limiting your total fat consumption to no more than 25-35% of total daily calories, with most coming from fish, nuts and vegetable oils. For a 2,000-calorie diet, that comes to 56-78 grams of fat a day. The AHA recommends a limit of 7% of daily calories from saturated fats, or 16 grams of saturated fat for a 2,000-calorie diet. Trans fats should comprise less than 1% of total daily calories, or less than 2 grams of trans fats a day on a 2,000-calorie diet. The FDA provides similar advice, recommending 65 grams of total fat, setting a limit of 20 grams of saturated fat and consuming as few trans fats as possible, based on a 2,000-calorie diet.

---

[32] *Katherine Zeratsky, R.D., L.D. "What does Percent Daily Value mean on food labels?" Mayo Clinic. 20 March 2025*
[33] *American Heart Association. "Know Your Fats." 21 April 2014*

Cholesterol and sodium should also be limited. The American Heart Association and the FDA recommend[34] limiting your cholesterol intake to 300mg a day, regardless of calorie intake. With regard to sodium, only a small amount occurs naturally in foods. Most of the sodium we consume is added during food processing, which is why our diet emphasizes fresh whole foods and minimizes the use of pre-made and processed foods. The DASH diet recommends[35] a daily limit of 2,300mg of sodium, which is very close to the FDA's recommendation of 2,400mg.

Vitamins and Minerals

Your goal should be to consume 100% of the recommended daily value of these key vitamins and minerals each day. Below are the recommendations by the U.S. FDA for several nutrients:

Nutrient	Amount
Vitamin A	5,000 International Units (IU)
Vitamin C	60mg
Thiamin	1.5mg
Riboflavin	1.7mg
Niacin	20mg
Calcium	1000mg
Iron	18mg
Vitamin D	400 IU
Vitamin E	30 IU
Vitamin B6	2mg
Folic acid	0.4mg
Vitamin B12	6 micrograms (mcg) (or 0.006 mg)
Phosphorus	1000mg
Iodine	150mcg (or 0.015mg)
Magnesium	400mg
Zinc	15mg
Copper	2mg
Biotin	0.3mg
Pantothenic acid	10mg

---

[34] *U.S. Food and Drug Administration. "How to Understand and Use the Nutrition Facts Label." 9 April 2015*
[35] *Heller, Maria. "Low Salt, Low Sodium and the DASH Diet." DASHDiet.org. 9 April 2015*

Chapter 21
Keep Stress Low

"Chronic stress is sometimes called "the silent killer" because it can damage both our physical health and our mental wellbeing. It is amazing to think that an overstressed mind can trigger health complications all throughout the body."

Now that you understand your diet and have made a plan, you will have to stay on that plan to achieve success. Change is hard! You will likely find that there are times when your new healthy habits do not seem worth it. Trips to the grocery store might seem more stressful as you try to decipher food labels and make healthier choices (especially in the beginning). Maybe you are unsure of how to navigate social situations now that you are trying to eat a healthier diet. Our food habits are deeply emotional (whether we realize it or not), and changing them can bring on unexpected emotional reactions. If you are going to successfully change your diet habits, you should understand that those feelings are normal. Do not let that stress get the best of you!

Chronic stress is sometimes called "the silent killer" because it can damage both our physical health and our mental wellbeing. Stress breaks down the order of our internal systems, frays our nerves, inhibits our immune system and disrupts our recovery from illnesses. It is amazing to think that an overstressed mind can trigger health complications all throughout the body.

Can Stress Affect GERD?

A 1999 survey of 2000 people attempted to find the answer to this question. The results of the study showed that individuals experienced heightened acid reflux symptoms after a tense day at work or during periods of significant family problems. A more recent study36 conducted in 2004 also supported the connection between GERD and stress. After a year of documenting GERD symptoms in sixty individuals, those with prolonged stress suffered greater amounts of heartburn episodes compared with those who were less stressed.

Tips for Managing Stress

Keeping stress under control is a very important part of maintaining your overall health. If you suffer from acid reflux, a plan to keep your mind at ease is paramount to acid reflux relief. More importantly, stress can also derail your diet program! Here are six things you can do to manage your stress and start relaxing.

---

[36] *Center for Neurovisceral Sciences & Women's Health, Department of Medicine, UCLA, Los Angeles, CA, USA. The effect of life stress on symptoms of heartburn. May 2004.*

Listen to Music

Music can quickly improve your mood. Experts know that there is a reason for playing music in elevators and while you are waiting on hold with your credit card company, and studies[37] have proven that it calms your mind and relaxes your body. Music can quickly get your thoughts off your worries. Listening to music that is upbeat helps to improve your mood with sounds that can lift your spirits. When you are working, cooking, cleaning or reading, for example, play music in order to stay positive. You will be surprised by the positive effect it has on you.

Make a Plan

Have you ever been stressed by the thought of unaccomplished tasks or overwhelmed by the large amounts of work yet to be done? "Getting your ducks in a row" can provide immediate relief from the burden of worry. Do not let an overdue task that you have procrastinated on fester in your mind. Prioritize your tasks, make a list and plan to follow it! Then get started, tackling each one in order. Once the plan is set, relieving the burden of this stress will feel like a physical weight has been lifted off your shoulders.

Meditate

Meditation sounds foreign and mysterious to some, but we encourage you to be open to this mental exercise. Meditation is simply a way to calm your mind. It is a conscious effort to quiet and rest your thoughts, allowing your mind to recalibrate and rebalance. Twenty minutes of meditation a day can be one of the most powerful weapons in our arsenal to combat stress. Many of those new to meditation are amazed by the clarity of mind than can follow a twenty-minute session. Meditation comes in many forms. We recommend exploring all options available to you. One easy and enjoyable technique is to simply lay down and listen to meditation music. Focus on the music and try to think of nothing else. You might find this to be more refreshing than a full night's sleep.

Laugh a Lot

Find a way to laugh. If you like movies, watch a comedy that you know and love. Spend time around fun light-hearted friends. Most importantly, laugh at yourself – it will give you much-needed levity. At the height of the Civil War, Abraham Lincoln sat down with his war council and opened up the meeting with a joke. An upset general rebuked him saying, "Mr. President, I don't think this is a time for laughter." Abraham Lincoln said, "General, if I cannot laugh, I should cry." Find a way to laugh.

---

[37] *Naliboff BD1, Mayer M, Fass R, Fitzgerald LZ, Chang L, Bolus R, Mayer EA.. "The effect of music on the human stress response." Center for Neurovisceral Sciences & Women's Health, Department of Medicine, UCLA, Los Angeles, CA, USA.*

Learn Something New

Pick up a subject that intrigues you and dive into it. Neurologists say that when we learn something new, it creates a new connection in our brain. Stress, on the other hand, can dull and kill these connections. One tool that may be used to combat this dullness is to engage in learning something fascinating, or pick up a new hobby. A mind that does not learn is a dormant mind, and it will soon find discouragement.

Exercise

Regular exercise is a great stress reliever. You will feel both physically and emotionally improved if you make exercise a regular part of your day. Exercise will increase the quantity neurotransmitters, known as endorphins, which send a message that says "I'm feeling good" to the brain. Exercise also takes your mind off of the very issues that create stress, resulting in a much clearer head and reduced stress levels.

Know Your Purpose

In Victor Frankl's book *A Man's Search For Meaning*, Frankl shares his experience in the Nazi internment camps and how it shaped him. He believes men who believed in purpose and those with a sense of personal destiny had the best chances of survival. A study done by the CDC[38] concluded that forty percent of Americans do not believe their lives have a purpose. Other research has shown[39] that people who believe their life has purpose have better outlooks on life, higher self-esteem, positive mental health, improved life satisfaction, improved resilience and less likelihood of depression. Examining your daily stresses within the context of your purpose can make them seem more manageable and easier to tackle.

[38] *Kobau, R., Sniezek, J., Zack, M. M., Lucas, R. E. and Burns, A. (2010), Well-Being Assessment: An Evaluation of Well-Being Scales for Public Health and Population Estimates of Well-Being among US Adults. Applied Psychology: Health and Well-Being, 2: 272–297. doi: 10.1111/j.1758-0854.2010.01035.x*

[39] *Hill PL1, Turiano NA2. Department of Psychology, Carleton University Department of Psychiatry, University of Rochester Medical Center, Rochester, New York. "Purpose in LIfe as a Predictor in Mortality across Adulthood." July 2014.*

Section IV
Diet Success: Successfully Making Behavioral Changes in Your Life

Introduction
Message from Michael R. Edelstein, Ph.D., Psychologist, Author, and Lecturer

"For the past thirty-five years I have been helping adults like you to change their lives dramatically for the better. I can honestly say, you can change dysfunctional behaviors that interfere with having a more satisfying and healthy life."

Building a Strategy to Succeed with Your Diet Program

Like many of you, a few years ago I noted symptoms in myself similar to those of acid reflux disease. As I began to research GERD, I found RefluxMD, a website devoted to helping people like you and me to create a plan for diagnosis, relief and good health. Not only was I able to learn a great deal about this chronic condition from the staff and medical advisors at RefluxMD, I also received detailed responses to many of my questions. Over time, I began a correspondence with several employees of RefluxMD and learned they were developing a diet program for GERD sufferers. They explained to me that although they were confident in their diet program for weight loss and GERD symptom relief, they were concerned that many of those starting their diet program would not succeed because they might fail to change their dietary behaviors. When they asked for my help, I was delighted – helping adults to tackle life's difficulties has been my life's work.

Knowing what to eat, how much and when is one thing – actually implementing it is quite another. This is the science of human behavioral change, or constructively addressing those behaviors that we know can actually hurt us. It is well established that excessive drinking is unhealthy and potentially life threatening, yet the WHO estimated[40] that 140 million adults have alcohol problems worldwide! Overeating and binge eating, smoking, and excessive alcohol consumption can all contribute to developing GERD, increasing the symptoms of this disease and hastening its progression. For those suffering from GERD, these behaviors can change…but how?

For the past thirty-five years I have been helping adults like you to change their lives dramatically for the better. I can honestly say, you can change dysfunctional behaviors that interfere with having a more satisfying and healthy life. This section will provide an overview of the principles and techniques that thousands have already used to positively change their lives. It is a self-help approach to managing life's emotional difficulties and correcting unhealthy behaviors. Some of you will understand these techniques after reading this section, but others may benefit from a more detailed explanation, which can be found in my book, *Three Minute Therapy*. For those who desire an individually

---

[40] *Riley, Leanne. "WHO to meet beverage company representative to discuss health-related alcohol issues." World Health Organization. 31 January 2003*

tailored approach, I invite you to contact me by phone or email.

As for my GERD story, I thank RefluxMD for their involvement and support. After trying several lifestyle changes and diet modifications, RefluxMD helped me to find a GERD expert who performed the necessary diagnostic tests to identify the underlying problem. RefluxMD's diet program is only one tool out of many that they offer to help you manage your disease and eliminate or reduce your symptoms. However, this diet program is very important in that it emphasizes diet and weight loss, the top recommendations by those who treat GERD. I encourage you to embrace this program with the confidence that the following concepts and strategies will keep you on the path to relief and good health.

Warm regards,
Michael

About Michael R. Edelstein, Ph.D.

Dr. Michael R. Edelstein is a practicing psychologist (in person, Skype, and via telephone therapy) in the San Francisco Bay Area who specializes in the treatment of anxiety, depression, relationship problems and addictions. He is the author of Three Minute Therapy, *a self-help book for overcoming common emotional and behavioral problems, for which he was awarded Author of the Year. Throughout his career, Dr. Edelstein has utilized Rational Emotive Behavior Therapy (REBT) approach to assist adults in making and mastering behavioral lifestyle changes, in pursuit of a happier life. With the simple yet powerful tools that he has created, Dr. Edelstein has successfully taught thousands of adults how to face difficulties in their lives and make lasting changes in the way they think, act, and feel. Other books published by Dr. Edelstein are Stage Fright, which includes interviews with Robin Williams, Jason Alexander, Melissa Etheridge, Maya Angelou and others, relating their personal experiences and wisdom in coping with performance anxiety; Rational Drinking: How to Live Happily With or Without Alcohol, which presents concepts, tools and strategies for overcoming compulsive drinking; and Therapy Breakthrough (with David Ramsey Steele and Richard Kujoth), a history and critique of the psychotherapy movement from Sigmund Freud to Albert Ellis. Dr. Edelstein was a training supervisor and fellow of the Albert Ellis Institute. He holds a diplomate in cognitive-behavioral therapy from the National Association of Cognitive-Behavioral Therapists, and is on its board of advisors. He was president of the Association for Behavioral and Cognitive Therapy. He is a certified sex therapist and has served as a consulting psychologist for the National Save-A-Life League, Inc., the oldest suicide prevention center in the United States. Dr. Edelstein was also a professional advisor to the San Francisco SMART Recovery Program. He was trained in REBT by Albert Ellis.*

Section IV: Diet Success
Successfully Making Behavioral Changes in Your Life

"Statements and thoughts that raise the emotional stakes in the world around us work their way into our minds insidiously, gradually, and without our knowing. They can be tremendous obstacles to our mental wellbeing as well as our ability to make positive changes in our lives. Affirming the belief that your thoughts control your feelings and emotions is a crucial step in controlling your destiny."

Overview

To effectively reduce or eliminate acid reflux symptoms, many people will make significant changes to their diet and lifestyle, and as eliminate some very entrenched and long-standing habits, specifically overeating, alcohol use and smoking. We recognize the challenge to overcome these behaviors and habits. Most successful adults use a working model or program to follow as they implement lifestyle changes. Therefore, psychological and behavioral instruction with corresponding tools to overcome these challenges contributes to success.

We were fortunate that Dr. Michael R. Edelstein approached RefluxMD with questions concerning acid reflux disease in 2014. As we got to know Dr. Edelstein, he shared many concepts about how to reduce or eliminate conscious or subconscious dysfunctional and destructive personal actions. Diets do not fail because of the quality or the amount of food, or because the dieter feels as if he is being deprived of something he wants, rather they fail because of poor thinking habits. Thanks to the principles presented by Dr. Edelstein, anyone beginning our GERD diet can remain sane and expect a high probability of success with the help of Dr. Edelstein's program.

To fortify dieters against expected periods of discouragement (which are bound to happen) it is vital to discuss the general concepts of overcoming adversity and understanding the root causes of why we fail to make personal lifestyle changes. The concepts presented by Dr. Edelstein not only address overcoming cravings, urges to eat and other dietary obstacles, but apply to a great many emotional and behavioral issues such as excessive drinking, smoking, anger, procrastination, panic attacks and anxiety as well.

Dr. Edelstein's discussion of why we fail to make positive lifestyle changes provides guidance to remedy the very common psychological obstacles that keep us from achieving our goals. In this section, we present the principles from Dr. Edelstein's book *Three Minute Therapy*, and we thank him for providing access and the opportunity to use sections of his book *Rational Drinking* for changing self-destructive habits.

Thinking Drives Emotion and Behavior

The fundamental principle that permeates this section is a simple truth: our feelings are a direct result of our thinking. However, it is important to clarify this is **NOT** a "think positive" methodology or one that teaches readers to picture "raindrops on roses and whiskers on kittens" just to brush off the occasional case of the "blues". This methodology teaches awareness of destructive thought habits – all too common in the minds of many people – as well as a way to overcome them. Many people fall victim to negative thoughts. It is essential, through a process called metacognition, to grow aware of negative self-fulfilling prophecies and deal with them accordingly.

Many of us do not realize it, but we are whiplashing our emotions around all day long, and most of the time, to the negative. Such common statements like, "Stupid drivers drive me crazy!" or, "Work deadlines are stressing me out!" are more harmful than we realize. When verbalized or even thought, these statements determine the degree of severity with which you will be affected by exterior circumstances. In essence, once you have a thought or made such a statement, this triggers your emotions. This inevitable event eventually occurs again and you respond accordingly with a predetermined level of severity.

Statements and thoughts that raise the emotional stakes in the world around us work their way into our minds insidiously, gradually, and without our knowing. They can be tremendous obstacles to our mental wellbeing as well as our ability to make positive changes in our lives. Affirming the belief that your thoughts control your feelings and emotions is a crucial step in controlling your destiny.

Debunking the Childhood Myth

Sigmund Freud, an Austrian neurologist who is known as the founding father of psychoanalysis, attempted to explain the reason why individuals can respond very differently to similar situations. By uncovering supposed traumatic childhood experiences, Freud believed he was able to explain a person's behavior, and that these childhood experiences cemented the way these people act today. Freud developed this theory in the late 19th and early 20th centuries, and ever since it has been the dominating psychological theme in the mind of the everyday person. This theory has caused many to scrutinize their parents and upbringing to find reasons for their shortcomings. Severely wounding the concept of self-responsibility, this theory often causes people to make their parents into scapegoats and victimize themselves.

There is absolutely no hard evidence that supports Freud's theory. Even when past childhood events affect a person in the present, it is not due to the event itself, but rather it is the individual's present belief about that memory that hurts the person – not the action itself.

Freud's theory is not only completely unsubstantiated, but it can be harmful to the person who believes it. It essentially robs the individual of the belief they are in control of their destiny and encourages a belief they are helpless in the face of past traumas too powerful to overcome. Removing any and all belief in popular misconceptions that contradict these realities is an essential step in moving forward and getting stronger.

Six Steps for Increasing Your Willpower

Many individuals who repeatedly fail to change their lives claim they lack willpower. This raises an important question: what is willpower?

Willpower is an ability we all have. The issue is whether we use it destructively or constructively. If you have bad habits, this means you have willfully developed and then stubbornly practiced these bad habits. Despite all the difficulties and red flags urging you to desist, you doggedly keep at it. This takes commitment, determination and willpower!

Once you have established the goal to stop or moderate your habits, redirect the will you have been using destructively into constructive thinking and acting. This involves a series of six steps. Let us examine each of them.

1. **Create a list of objectives**. Do you want to quit or start something, or is this a more moderate desire? If the latter is true, specify in detail what your moderation will consist of, i.e. eliminate soda pop completely or allow one can of soda every week.

2. **Decide when you will make this change**. This step involves recognizing your desire and your ability to succeed. On its own, the desire alone is not enough. Wishing to stop and setting a date does not mean you will act on it. The next four steps will help to turn your desire into action.

3. **Find the determination to change your habits**. Resolve that no matter what, you will do whatever it takes to achieve your goals, with no excuses and no debates!

4. **Learn what you can about disciplining your habits and how to overcome your urges**. Seek out cognitive, emotive and behavioral ways to reach your goal. (Reading the rest of this section will be a great start!) Then practice, practice, practice.

5. **Take action**. Stick to your plan. If you have decided to quit something altogether, then stop doing it now.

6. **Have a plan to deal with backsliding**. It is not easy to change, and you may often take missteps and return to your old ways. But you are prepared because you recognize, like everyone else on the planet, you are a fallible human being who often makes mistakes. You know learning frequently involves two steps forward and one step back. You do not let that deter you. You are determined to succeed, so instead of abandoning your goal when you have lapsed, you resolve not to give up.

Using your willpower constructively means changing your thinking and taking action; it means working hard to reinforce new habits and refusing to give in to failure. You may dream of easy ways to achieve your goals, but they do not exist. Unfortunately in life, meaningful gains are rarely achieved without pain.

A Little-Known Fact About Why We Fail at Self-Improvement

The main reason people eat unhealthy foods, smoke or drink to excess is to satisfy an urge, and the underlying motivation for satisfying an urge is to feel good. Even though these things may make you feel worse later, there is a powerful temptation that resurfaces over and over again, pressing us into committing these acts.

We have also seen it is human nature to want to avoid unpleasant feelings and to seek out good feelings. People who have failed at self-improvement in the past often go one step further: they insist – **they demand** – that they must avoid all unpleasant feelings in order to only have good feelings.

The reason why you fail to resist your vices is because you believe you *must* feel better or escape discomfort. You have escalated your already strong desire to feel good into a *demand* to feel good and escape discomfort. This thinking is at the root of what has driven you to succumb to your temptations.

Long-Term vs. Short-Term Happiness

Most people want to be happy. We want to be happy when we are by ourselves, when we are with others – especially when we are with our significant others – when we are at work or school, and during our leisure time.

We are quite resourceful in finding ways to make ourselves happy. We can do it in simple ways such as by listening to music, watching a movie or play, or going to a sporting event. Or we can do it in more creative ways such as by building a yacht and sailing around the world, writing a book, getting a postgraduate degree, or training to run a marathon.

Some forms of happiness can be acquired quite quickly and easily while others take time and effort. Both ways of seeking happiness are legitimate and each has its place in our lives.

Sometimes in our quest to find short-term (quick and easy) happiness, we sabotage our goal of long-term happiness. For example, if you spend all of your disposable income going to concerts and movies, this may mean forfeiting your goal to see the world, since you have no money left over for travel.

Similarly, if you were to eat frequently and copiously in a quest to find short-term happiness, you may damage your health and risk losing any chance of leading a long and healthy life.

You risk your long-term happiness when you insist – demand – that you **must** be happy right now, even if that means missing out on what you want in the long run.

Here is how it works. You begin with a desire to get rid of bad feelings and replace them with good feelings. Then you escalate your desire for good feelings into a demand for the good feelings you get from overeating, excessive drinking, or smoking by convincing yourself you **absolutely need** to do one of these activities. Do this often enough and sooner or later your short-term indulgence destroys any hope you have for long-term happiness.

If you are like most people, you have a goal to lead a long, healthy, happy life. This may be the most important goal you will ever have. By overeating, smoking or drinking excessively, you replace what you desire most with what you tell yourself you **must** have right now. In other words, it is your view – your belief – in the **need** for short-term escape that ultimately destroys your chances of long-term happiness. Going for short-term happiness compulsively sabotages deep satisfaction and fulfillment in life.

Five Signs of Self-Defeating Thinking

Human beings often act quite sanely. This keeps us alive. If we were not reasonable, we would not have the good sense to eat our bread when we are hungry, pay bills when they are due and find relationships when we are lonely.

As realistic as we are, we can also act quite crazily, often behaving in ways that interfere with our short- and long-term health and happiness. For example, we get angry at our car or computer when it does not run smoothly, despite the fact that machines have no way of detecting or responding to our rage. We put off going to see the doctor or dentist even though it is in our best interests to see them as scheduled. And, of course, we often overeat, drink excessively, and smoke more copiously than is good for us.

More often than not, our self-defeating behavior is caused by ignorance or irrational beliefs. Irrational beliefs usually have one or more of the following characteristics:

1. Although irrational beliefs may seem true and sensible to us at the time, upon closer examination it is quite easy to see they are false and nonsensical.
2. They often lead us to thinking less of ourselves and putting ourselves down as unworthy human beings.
3. They interfere with our relationships, making it difficult for us to get along with others.
4. They make us sedentary and unproductive.
5. They prevent us from reaching our short-term – and more frequently our long-term – goals.

So where do these irrational beliefs come from?

For the most part, we are born with the tendency to overgeneralize, condemn and absolutize. These irrational proclivities appear across all cultures and throughout all of history. None of us are immune to them. Even psychologists, whom you might think would know better, are prone to them.

Further evidence we are born with this unreasonable proclivity comes from the observation despite our best efforts to act reasonably, unaffected by irrational thinking; we often continue to resort to self-defeating behavior. Additionally, we continue to act in self-defeating ways even though our friends and family frown upon our actions, and even when we dislike our own behavior.

In addition to being born with a tendency to subscribe to irrational beliefs, our culture, media, parents, teachers and friends often reinforce our irrational beliefs. They sometimes tell us such nonsense as, "You **must** do this and you **must** not do that, and if you do otherwise you are a failure."

The greatest influencing factor by far, which leads us to cling to our irrational beliefs, is our own self-talk. We constantly reinforce our irrational beliefs, telling ourselves the same old nonsense over and over: "I **must** eat this pizza," or "I **need** to get a drink right now," or "I really **need** a smoke!" In other words, we say to ourselves: "I **must** get the good feelings from (insert activity), and I **must** get them right now or else life is **terrible** and **I cannot stand it**."

Seven Questions to Drive You Sane

As we have already seen, your struggle to quit or cut down on certain habits is sabotaged by irrational beliefs are standing between you and your goals. These beliefs include the idea you *have to* get rid of bad feelings and replace them with the good feelings you get from overeating, drinking to excess or smoking.

A constructive war on these forces begins with a battle with these destructive beliefs. The strategy for destroying these beliefs involves four steps:

1. Identify the irrational beliefs that interfere with your happiness, such as "I *absolutely must* satisfy my urge right now!"

2. Once you have identified these beliefs, question and challenge them. This means searching for supporting evidence for these notions. Ask yourself, "What is the evidence that shows I absolutely *must* (rather than strongly prefer to) satisfy my urge?"

3. Prove to yourself your thinking is false, nonsensical and destructive. In particular, convince yourself it is not a *necessity* to rid yourself of bad feelings and have only good feelings. Show yourself this belief makes no sense and is destructive. Reinforce the notion there are no *musts, shoulds, have tos* or *dire necessities*. You do not run the universe, so nothing *has to* be your way. You do not have perfect control over your body, mind, feelings or circumstances, so an ideal state is never in the cards, although it would be lovely if it were.

4. As you uproot your addictive thinking, reinforce constructive beliefs that are realistic, logical and pragmatic (i.e. they aid you in achieving better self-control). Practice telling yourself you can survive quite well if you do not give in to the pleasure of the moment. Further, convince yourself you can bear facing discomfort – even great discomfort – without overeating, drinking or smoking.

Proving to yourself the beliefs leading to any of these bad habits are false is the most important step. It is the vital key to controlling your life. You can show yourself your goal-sabotaging beliefs are false, illogical and destructive by challenging them with these key questions:

1. Is this idea consistent with the facts? Is it true?

2. What evidence is there for the falsehood of this belief?

3. Does this idea follow consistently from my values and preferences? Is it logical?

4. Does this idea help me to reach my long-term goals? Is it pragmatic?

5. What are better alternative ideas that are realistic, logical and pragmatic?

6. What is the worst that is likely to happen if I do not get what I think I must? The likely worst-case scenario if I do not drown my bad feelings in eating, drinking or smoking is I will feel bad for a while! I may not enjoy the party as much or fit in as well with my friends, but as we saw earlier, "No pain, no gain!"

7. What are some positive things that could happen – or I could make happen – if I do not get what I think I **must**? I could beat my alcohol, eating or smoking addiction, eliminate uncomfortable cravings, feel healthier, improve my relationships and increase my productivity at work.

Utilizing the answers to these seven key questions will result in a more rational attitude toward your problems. This will help you cut down or quit your alcohol consumption, smoking and overeating, and will help you to reach your long-term health goals.

The ABCs of Rational Thinking

The ideas in this section are based on the teachings of Dr. Albert Ellis who created a brand-new type of psychotherapy in 1955, now known as Rational Emotive Behavior Therapy, or REBT. REBT was the first cognitive behavioral therapy, and has proven to be effective in treating a large number of emotional and behavioral problems including alcohol and smoking dependence as well as overeating.

Albert Ellis developed a simple ABC model, which he used to teach his clients how to be their own therapists. In this model, A stands for the Activating event – the situation you were in or the feeling you had before you started overeating; B stands for your unhelpful irrational Beliefs about the activating event; and C stands for the Consequences of combining A with B. Here is how it works:

A. (Activating event): Something happens or you have a particular thought or feeling.

B. (Irrational beliefs): You have a demand – a **must, should** or **have to**.

C. (Consequences): You react to the situation in an unhelpful way.

When it comes to sabotaging your long-term health goals by eating excessively, the ABC model looks like this:

A. (Activating event): I want to replace the bad feelings I have with the good feelings I get from eating.

B. (Beliefs): I **must** feel better. I **need** to eat.

C. (Consequences): Binge eating.

As you can see from the ABC model presented above, it is not your urge (A) to replace your bad feelings with good feelings that causes you to overeat, it is your beliefs (B) that lead to undesirable consequences (C).

Imagine how this might look if you held rational rather than irrational beliefs at point B:
A. (Activating event): I want to replace my bad feelings with the good feelings I get from eating.
B. (Rational beliefs): I would like eat more and feel better, but I do not **need** to feel better and I certainly do not **need** to eat more.
C. (Consequences): Refrain from binge eating.

By using the ABC model to change your beliefs, you may change the outcome! When you convince yourself you do not **need** to eat more, you may more easily keep your urges in check.

When it comes to changing your eating habits and reaching your long-term goals, the ABC model is your best friend.

How to Control Your Thinking in Three Minutes

The ABC model clearly demonstrates the role your beliefs play in your response to your urges. It becomes an even more powerful tool for change when you expand it to include points D, E and F.

In this expanded model, D stands for Disputing or questioning the irrational Beliefs; E stands for an Effective new way of thinking; and F stands for your new Feelings and behaviors.

At point D, you challenge the beliefs you identified at point B by asking "Why?" or "What is the evidence for my **must**?" For example, "Why **must** I have a drink right now?" At point E you answer this question with effective new perspectives, which aids you in achieving your goals. At point F you describe how you feel and how you will respond when you subscribe to the new way of thinking.

Let us look at an example to illustrate how this process might work for you:
A. (Activating event): I want to replace the bad feelings I have with the good feelings I get from drinking.
B. (Irrational beliefs): I **must** feel better right now. I **need** a drink.
C. (Consequences): Drinking.
D. (Disputing or questioning): Why **must** I feel better right now? What is the evidence I **need** a drink?

E. (Effective new thinking): As much as I would like to replace my bad feelings with the good feelings I get from alcohol, there is no law indicating I *must* replace these feelings. It is not true I *need* a drink. Similarly, just because I want to drink, it does not logically follow that I *must* have one or I *need* one. The idea that I *must* feel better and I *need* a drink leads to behavior that is ultimately self-destructive and sabotages my long-term health, relationships and financial goals. It would be far better for me to convince myself of the alternative idea, although I would like a drink, I definitely do not *need* one. It is preferable for me to find more constructive means to achieve happiness than through excessive alcohol consumption.

F. (New feeling and behavior): I feel uncomfortable going without a drink, but by convincing myself of the new philosophy, I may successfully abstain.

By regularly writing this expanded ABCDEF model – once or more, every day – you will conquer your old habits and replace them with new patterns in line with your long-term goals. Once you have had practice using this exercise, it will only take a few minutes to complete it. This is why we call it the Three Minute Exercise (TME).

Study the TMEs that follow to help you gain a complete and thorough understanding of how to overcome your bad habits and negative thought patterns, and reach your long-term health goals.

How to Stop Beating Yourself Up

Perhaps you are one of the many people who fall off the diet wagon and then beat yourself up for it. There is a better way. Instead of despairing, you can avoid creating these problems in the first place with the TME.

A. (Activating event): I smoked a pack of cigarettes last night.

B. (Beliefs): I *should not* have smoked so much. I am *worthless*.

C. (Consequences): I feel worthless and ashamed, and will smoke again to drown my bad feelings.

D. (Disputing or questioning): Why *should I not* have smoked so much? Where is the evidence I am worthless?

E. (Effective new thinking): I have made a decision to cut down on my smoking. However, it is not compulsory for me to smoke less, it is a choice. There is no reason why I *absolutely must* stop smoking or smoke less. Acting against my own best wishes does not magically make me worthless. While my actions are unwise and foolish, my worth as a human being never varies – it does not go up and down based on how much or how little I smoke. My choice to cut down on smoking does not mean I *absolutely must* stop smoking or cut down on it, although I passionately desire to do so. Nor does it logically follow because I smoked more than I had initially intended, I become a failure as a person. Putting myself down for smoking only makes me feel bad about myself, which often leads me to smoke even more. Therefore, telling myself I am *worthless* does not help me to reach my long-term goals – instead, it makes it harder for me to reach them. Rather than telling myself I ***should not*** have smoked so much and I am *worthless* because I did, I had better convince myself smoking is a choice and I am determined to succeed at smoking less, no matter how many setbacks I have along the way. It would be better for me to decide and re-decide to abstain rather than giving up. Instead of convincing myself I am *worthless* for having smoked more than I intended, it would be more useful for me to accept the fact I am a fallible human being who will sometimes act against my own best interests. Such actions do not make me worthless. Success involves learning from my mistakes and often going one step back with every two steps forward.

F. (New feeling and behavior): I feel quite disappointed I smoked so much, but not worthless and filled with self-loathing. Stick to my original decision to cut down on my smoking.

Get into the habit of using the TME to overcome any feelings of shame or self-loathing you have after smoking, drinking excessively, overeating or falling off your diet plan. Even more importantly, practice writing out the TMEs daily in preparation for tempting situations that arise unexpectedly. Using this model consistently will make it much easier for you to avoid these temptations as a means for drowning your bad feelings.

Make Allowances for Setbacks

In the example below, a man on a diet has fallen off for the first time.

A. The fact or situation: I cheated on my diet.

B. Your unreasonable "musty" subconscious belief: I **must** never cheat on my diet. This proves I am a failure.

C. Your reaction: I feel like a loser and a failure. I'm giving up on my diet.

The result is a loss of confidence and declining commitment to the goal of dieting. In this case, then add parts D, E and F, recording and analyzing inner dialogue that will help you to think rationally about your setback.

D. Dispute and question the merits of Step B: Where is it etched in stone I **must** never cheat on my diet? Is it really possible to never cheat? Does one instance of cheating prove I am a failure?

E. The enlightened new thinking about Step B: I wish I had not cheated on my diet, but since I am human and imperfect, of course I will screw up at times. I do not magically turn into a total failure when I screw up. It is frustrating to experience a setback, but it is hardly the end of the universe. Condemning myself for backsliding does not help and only makes things worse. With practice and reinforcement, I can learn to unconditionally accept my imperfect behavior and myself.

F. Your new reaction to cheating on your diet: I did slip up, but succeeding is important to me. Although I may slip up occasionally, I am determined to keep working at it and succeed in the long run.

By regularly thinking through this enlightened new philosophy, you will become emotionally settled with a new mindset for a quicker rebound, which will lead to a greater success rate.

Getting on with Getting it Right

The purpose of this section has been to teach you powerful concepts and tools that will help you to achieve your identified goals on your path to relief from GERD symptoms. It does not tell you what your objective should be. It does not insist you either stop or moderate your habits. It is up to you to choose the most reasonable approach for you to live a better life.

Whether your goal is to reduce the amount of calories you eat, the frequency with which you drink, or quit smoking altogether, you now know how to achieve a realistic mindset for success. Just as it is up to you to choose your goal, it is up to you how much you will use these tools to reach your goals. You will be happier and more productive if you are motivated by strong preferences rather than by absolute demands. Your likelihood of success will be greatly enhanced if you employ the practical, rational steps described, all the while being aware there is no guarantee of immediate success. Have patience and take a long-term perspective. Face discomfort now for the purpose of achieving more comfort in the long run.

In this section, a limited number of the most common reasons people fail at making desired changes in their life were described, as well as some specific examples of ways to employ the TME. It is possible your particular rationalizations or circumstances were not mentioned. However, a wonderful feature of the TME lies in its adaptability, enabling you to meet your personal requirements for success.

The TME puts you in charge of your life. In effect, by practicing the TME you may reduce or eliminate the usefulness of attending self-help groups or therapy. You act as your own therapist!

It is important to recognize all of the exercises presented are designed to be done daily in preparation for tempting situations. Practice these tools religiously and make it second nature to do so.

In addition, the learning process is often comprised of progress mixed with lapses. You will ultimately succeed if you refuse to give up in the face of setbacks. Most individuals who overcome their compulsive habits do not expect immediate or perfect success. Rather, it is those who become adamantly determined to persevere, no matter how difficult the bumps are along the way, who ultimately succeed. Work and practice, work and practice: these are the keys to overcoming most of life's difficulties.

If you require expert assistance or counseling, please contact Dr. Michael R. Edelstein at (415) 673-3848 or email him at DrEdelstein@ThreeMinuteTherapy.com. Dr. Edelstein offers clinical psychology sessions via phone, Skype and in person.

Section V
Meal Plans

21-Day Meal Plans

"RefluxMD's 21 daily meal plans are designed to give you structure. It maintains the necessary integrity of the DASH diet, but also allows flexibility in meal planning. These daily meal plans are also GERD-friendly."

Following a diet plan can sometimes get complicated, so we designed 21 easy to follow daily meal plans to aid you in your endeavor. The RefluxMD daily meal plans will serve as a roadmap to help you meet your personal needs and food preferences. *RefluxMD's Recipe for Relief* was developed using the #1 rated DASH diet, which was created by the National Institute of Health to reduce high blood pressure. The DASH diet also proved to be highly effective as a balanced, safe and healthy weight loss program. In fact, the DASH diet earned the "TOP DIET" award for five consecutive years from US News and World Report after expert evaluations of over 35 diets. Other diets rated in the study include Weight Watchers (#3), Jenny Craig (#8), and Atkins (#29).

Based upon these convincing results, RefluxMD selected the DASH diet as the foundation for its *Recipe for Relief*. Since the DASH diet was not specifically formulated for those with GERD, RefluxMD designed meal plans that avoid known trigger foods, and created over 90 recipes to meet the needs of those suffering from acid reflux disease.

NIH DASH Diet Design

When RefluxMD first looked at the DASH diet, it seemed complex. However, after a more detailed review, we realized that its effectiveness is based upon three primary factors:

Calories per day

Based upon each individual's goals, calories can range from 1,600 calories per day to 2,400 calories per day, or even higher based upon activity levels. Serving sizes can be increased or decreased to accommodate an individual's targeted calorie level.

Sodium per day

The DASH diet's guideline for sodium consumption is between 1,500 milligrams to 2,400 milligrams per day. However, since active adults can lose sodium during physical activity, RefluxMD's 21-day meal plan uses a range of 1,600 to 2,600 milligrams of sodium. Again, adjustments can be easily made to achieve alternative sodium levels.

DASH food groups per day

Good health requires balance in the types of foods consumed so that your body gets the nutrition it needs. For GERD sufferers, that means not only watching how much you eat, but also what you eat as well. The NIH DASH diet recommends a specific number of food servings from key food groups based upon the targeted daily calorie consumption.

An illustration of how food groups are incorporated into the DASH diet is highlighted below:

NIH Recommend Food Servings Daily

Food Group Equivalent = 1 food group	1,600 Calorie Diet	2,600 Calorie Diet
Grains *1 slice bread; ½ cup cooked pasta, rice, or cereal; ¼ bagel; 1 oz. dry cereal; ½ English muffin, bun; 2 cups popcorn; 2 small cookies.*	6	10 - 11
Vegetables *1 cup raw leafy vegetable, ½ up cut-up raw or cooked vegetable, ½ cup vegetable juice.*	3 – 4	5 - 6
Fruits ½ cup juice, 1 medium fruit, ¼ cup dried fruit, ½ cup fresh, frozen or canned fruit, 1 cup diced raw fruit.	4	5 - 6
Low Fat Diary *1 cup skim or low-fat milk, 1 cup low-fat/fat- free yogurt, 1 oz. reduced-fat cheese, ½ cup fat-free or low-fat cottage cheese.*	2 - 3	3
Lean Meats, Poultry, Fish and Eggs 1 oz. cooked meat, poultry or fish, *1 egg = 1 oz.*, 2 *egg whites = 1 oz.*	3 - 6	6
Nuts, Seeds, and Legumes *1/3 cup or 1.5 oz. of beans, nuts, seeds; 2 tbsp. peanut butter; 2 tbsp. or .5 oz. of seeds; .5 cup of cooked legumes (dried beans, peas, etc.).*	1/2	1

Using RefluxMD's Program - Daily Meal Plans

Managing the consumption of calories, sodium, and six food groups requires some structure. RefluxMD's 21 daily meal plans are designed to give you that structure. It maintains the necessary integrity of the DASH diet, but also allows flexibility in meal planning. These daily meal plans are also GERD-friendly. RefluxMD' diet program offers daily meal plans that include a breakfast, a morning snack, a lunch, an afternoon snack, and dinner. Each daily meal plan is identified by the primary lunch and dinner entre in the title, and each plan is categorized as "Low Caloric" (1,600 – 1,900 calories),

"Moderate Caloric" (1,901 – 2,300 calories), or "High Caloric" (2,301 – 2,600 calories). The example below is the second day from the moderate calorie week:

Moderate Caloric - Day 2
Grilled Mushroom Quesadilla / Filet Mignon
2,237 C – 2,032 S

Breakfast - 600 C / 673 S
Corn Flakes with Milk, Bagel with Cream Cheese and Peach Nectar
Cereal, corn flakes (2/3 cup) with milk, fat free (.5 cup)
Bagel, cinnamon-raisin (med) with cream cheese, low fat (2T)
Peach nectar (1 cup)

Morning Snack - 215 C / 1 S
Pineapple Slices with Almonds
Pineapple (2 slices)
Almonds (.3 cup)

Lunch - 674 C / 833 S
Grilled Mushroom Quesadilla with Sweet Potato Fries and an Apple
Grilled Mushroom Quesadilla **RMD** (1 serving) with sweet potato fries [Ore Ida] (3 oz.)
Apple (medium)

Afternoon Snack - 160 C / 285 S
Cheddar Cheese and Sourdough Pretzels
Cheese, lite cheddar [Laughing Cow](1 wedge)
Pretzels, sourdough [Snyder's] (20 mini pretzels)

Dinner – 588 C / 240 S
Filet Mignon and Mushrooms with a Baked Potato, Asparagus, a Dinner Roll and Peaches
Filet Mignon, barbequed or baked (3 oz.) with mushrooms, sliced (3 oz.)
Baked potato (medium) with butter, unsalted (1T)
Asparagus, cooked (.5 cup)
Roll, whole-wheat (small)
Peaches (.5 cup)

DASH Servings: 8 grain, 5.8 vegetables, 5.5 fruit, 3.6 dairy, 3 meat/fish/poultry, 1 nuts/seeds

C = calories, S = sodium in mg., (#t) = teaspoons, (#T) = tablespoons, RMD = RefluxMD recipe that can be found in the recipe section, [name] = food manufacturer brand

Tips Before You Get Started

Be patient and take your time
Most adults today consume more than 2,600 calories and more than 2,600 milligrams of sodium daily. If that sounds like you, be sure to start slowly and begin with our high caloric daily meal plans. This will allow you to become comfortable with the meal planning process as you transition into fewer calories and less sodium over time. Think of this as a marathon rather than a 100-yard dash.

Look for recipes, foods, and snacks that you enjoy
You should enjoy the foods that you eat, even on a diet or when following a meal plan. Find recipes and other foods you enjoy and write down their caloric and sodium levels. As you become more effective at daily and weekly planning, you can swap in these foods to balance your program.

Commit to maintain a balanced diet
Managing calories and sodium consumption is essential, however you should also manage the quantities of the DASH food groups for proper nutrition. Hitting the exact daily target is ideal, but there is some wiggle room here. It is fine to be plus-or-minus one food serving of the daily target on occasion.

Portion size is important
If you use RefluxMD's recommended portions, please attempt to stay within the specified amounts. For example, 20 Snyder mini pretzels provide the correct amount of calories and sodium, and equals one grain serving. Many of the foods and snacks we suggest are tasty, and you may want to consume more. However, you should try to eat the amounts recommended in the daily meal plans.

Experiment by substituting meals and snacks into other days
Changing it up will not only keep your interest, but it may prove to be more enjoyable as well. RefluxMD posted the calories and sodium in each meal and snack, making it easy to take the entire section to create a new daily plan. This will become clear to you and easy to do once you get started with *Recipe for Relief.*

Make a shopping list and keep your pantry stocked
Every day requires grains, vegetables, dairy products, and meat, poultry or fish servings. To succeed with this meal program you will need to have several of these food groups available daily. Be sure to stock up on each food group when you shop for groceries to keep your diet balanced and healthy.

Use RefluxMD's GERD-friendly recipes

We have inserted our recipes into the daily meal plans to highlight them for you, and in some cases there are several of our recipes in a single daily meal plan. These are recommendations, but we also realize that cooking and preparation time may be limited. Again, they are included as examples for your benefit and we hope that you enjoy them.

Caution when substituting your favorite recipes, foods or snacks

Before you use one of your favorite recipes, spend a few moments computing both the calories and the sodium in the ingredients. For example, the Zappa Family Spaghetti Sauce recipe (printed in the NYT) has 481 calories and 1,893 mg of sodium per serving! It also contains several known GERD triggers including onions, garlic, tomatoes, and tomato sauce. Yes, it is a family favorite with the Zappa family, but for those with GERD, it will hinder your diet and potentially trigger your acid reflux symptoms.

Finally, we hope that you enjoy these meal plans and our recipes and that you make them part of your diet program. Personal taste and food preferences are very different among adults, but we hope that we have offered you a variety of recipes and plans that will assist you on your path to relief and good health.

Summary of RefluxMD's Daily Meal Plans

The daily meal plan titles highlight the lunch, dinner, number of calories (C) and amount of sodium (S) in milligrams.

High Caloric Daily Meal Plans – 2,301 to 3,000 Calories
Day 1 ~ Chicken Pita / Mustard Pork Loin ~ 2,882 C ~ 2,490 S
Day 2 ~ Turkey Sandwich / Chicken Cheese Bake ~ 2,676 C ~2,430 S
Day 3 ~ Vegetable Chowder / Tuna Casserole ~ 2,608 C ~ 2,361 S
Day 4 ~ Lentil Burger / Beef Mushroom Skillet ~ 2,571 C ~ 2,125 S
Day 5 ~Chicken Salad Sandwich / Beef Eye Round ~ 2,503 C ~ 1,638 S
Day 6 ~ Shrimpy Spinach Salad / Stuffed Port Tenderloin ~ 2,415 C ~ 2,431 S
Day 7 ~ Veggy Mac and Cheese / Pasta Primavera ~ 2,305 C ~ 2,055 S

Moderate Caloric Daily Meal Plans – 1,901 to 2,300 Calories
Day 1 ~ Split Pea Soup / Chicken and Dumplings ~ 2,255 C ~ 2,069 S
Day 2 ~ Grilled Mushroom Quesadilla / Filet Mignon ~ 2,237 C ~ 2,031 S
Day 3 ~ Egg Salad Sandwich / Fish Tacos ~ 2,144 C ~ 1,696 S
Day 4 ~ Lentil Burger / Baked Halibut ~ 2,142 C ~ 1,930 S
Day 5 ~ Turkey Burger / Gingersnap Beef Stew ~ 2,127 C ~ 1,744 S
Day 6 ~ Tuna Melt / Curry Almond Chicken ~ 1,983 C ~ 2,050 S
Day 7 ~ Chicken Sandwich / Tuna Casserole ~ 1,927 C ~ 2,313 S

Low Caloric Daily Meal Plans – 1,600 to 1,900 Calories

Day 1 ~ Chicken Pita / Fish in Parchment ~ 1,862 C ~ 1,660 S

Day 2 ~ Cobb Salad / Braised Short Ribs ~ 1,839 C ~ 2,193 S

Day 3 ~ Chicken Quesadilla / Mustard Pork Loin ~ 1,829 C ~ 2,189 S

Day 4 ~ Chicken Salad / Oven Steamed Tilapia ~ 1,837 C ~ 1,402 S

Day 5 ~ Grilled Cheese / Shrimp and Pea Stir Fry ~ 1,769 C ~ 2,117

Day 6 ~ Vegetable and White Bean Soup / Roasted Salmon ~ 1,715 C ~ 1,686 S

Day 7 ~ Shrimp Pita / Vegetable Chowder ~ 1,638 C ~ 1,799 S

Daily Meal Plans

The abbreviations used in the daily meal plans are:

C = calories, S = sodium in mg., (#t) = teaspoons, (#T) = tablespoons, RMD = RefluxMD recipe that can be found in the recipe section, [name] = food manufacturer brand

High Caloric Daily Meal Plans – 2,301 to 3,000 Calories

High Caloric - Day 1
Chicken Pita / Mustard Pork Loin
2,882 C – 2,490 S

Breakfast - 723 C / 488 S
Oats, Nuts and Berries with Toast, Jam and Grape Juice
Oats, Nuts, and Berry Breakfast **RMD** (1 cup)
Bread, white, toasted (2 slices) with jam or jelly [Smuckers] – (1T)
Grape Juice (1 cup)

Morning Snack - 528 C / 524 S
Cinnamon-Raisin Bagel with Cream Cheese, a Banana and Milk
Bagel, cinnamon-raisin (1 medium) with cream cheese, low fat (2T)
Banana (medium)
Milk, fat free (1 cup)

Lunch - 552 C / 624 S
Chicken Pita with Whole Wheat Crackers and a Banana
Pita bread, wheat (regular); chicken, cooked and cubed (2 oz.); yogurt, no fat [Chobani]; lettuce, shredded (1 oz.); garbanzo beans (1 oz.); olives, green; and diced (2 olives)
Crackers, whole wheat (6 pcs)
Apple (med)

Afternoon Snack - 422 C / 237 S
Granola Cereal Snack with Milk and Grapes
Cereal, granola [Open Nature] (.5 cup)
Grapes (.5 cup)
Milk, fat free (1 cup)

Dinner – 657 C / 617 S
Mustard Pork Loin, Green Beans, Baked Potato with Sour Cream, Diner Roll w/Butter
Mustard Pork Loin **RMD** (4 oz.)
Potato baked (large) with low-fat sour cream (1T)
Roll, whole wheat (small) with unsalted butter (1t)

DASH Servings: 10 grain, 5 vegetables, 6 fruit, 3.8 dairy, 6 meat/fish/poultry, 0 nuts/seeds

High Caloric - Day 2
Turkey Sandwich / Chicken Cheese Bake
2,676 C / 2,430 S

Breakfast - 626 C / 635 S
Oatmeal with Raisins, Bagel with Cream Cheese, and Milk
Oatmeal, instant (.5 cup) with raisins (.3 cup)
Bagel, whole wheat (large) with low fat cream cheese (1T)
Milk, fat free (1 cup)

Morning Snack - 649 C / 102 S
Fruit Yogurt, Walnuts and a Banana
Yogurt, low fat with fruit (6 oz.)
Walnuts (2 oz.)
Banana (medium)

Lunch - 423 C / 909 S
Turkey Sandwich, Potato Salad, Carrots, and Fruit Cocktail
Turkey, low sodium [Columbus] (2 oz.); romaine lettuce (1 leaf); bread, whole wheat (2 slices); Dijon mustard (1t)
Carrots (.5 cup)
Picnic Potato Salad **RMD**, .5 cup

Afternoon Snack – 176 C / 147 S
Crackers with an Apple
Crackers, whole wheat (6 pieces)
Apple (medium)

Dinner – 712 C / 512 S
Chicken Cheese Bake, Corn, White Rice, Cantaloupe, Dinner Roll, Strawberry Jello, Milk
Chicken Cheese Bake **RMD** (1 cup) with rice, white medium grain, (.5 cup), and corn (.5 cup)
Roll, whole-wheat dinner (small) with margarine, soft (1t)
Jell-O [Spangles] (6 oz.)
Milk, fat free (1 cup)

DASH Servings: 9 grain, 4.25 vegetables, 5 fruit, 3 dairy, 4 meat/fish/poultry, 2 nuts/seeds

High Caloric - Day 3
Vegetable Chowder / Tuna Casserole
2,608 C – 2,361 S

Breakfast - 577 C / 330 S
Scrambled Eggs, Toast with Jelly and Pineapple Juice
Eggs, scrambled (2 eggs) with milk, fat free (1T)
Bread, white and toasted (2 slices); margarine soft (1T); and jelly/ jam [Smucker's] (1T)
Pineapple juice (1 cup)

Morning Snack - 395 C / 126 S
Frosted Wheat Cereal with Milk and a Banana
Cereal, frosted wheat [Fiber One] (1 cup) with milk, fat free (1 cup)
Banana (medium)

Lunch – 407 C / 903 S
Vegetable Chowder with a Roll and Apple Juice
Vegetable Chowder *RMD* (1 cup)
Roll, whole-wheat (small) with margarine (1t)
Apple juice (.5 cup)

Afternoon Snack - 500 C / 358 S
Peanut Butter Milkshake. Triscuits Crackers, and Grapes
Peanut Butter Milkshake RMD (1 cup)
Triscuits (12 crackers)
Grapes (.5 cup)

Dinner – 729 C / 644 S
Tuna Casserole, Garden Salad, Peaches, Coconut Rice Pudding, and Milk
Tuna Casserole *RMD* (1 cup)
Lettuce, iceberg (1 cup); cumbers, sliced (.25 cup); carrots, shredded (.3 cup); topped
  with Apricot Vinaigrette Dressing *RMD* (2T)
Peaches (.5 cup)
Milk, fat free (1 cup)
Coconut Rice Pudding *RMD* (.5 cup)

DASH Servings: 10 grain, 5 vegetables, 6.25 fruit, 3.5 dairy, 4 meat/fish/poultry, 1 nuts/seeds

High Caloric - Day 4
Lentil Burger / Beef Mushroom Skillet
2,571 C – 2,125 S

Breakfast - 339 C / 191 S
Sweet Vanilla Smoothie with a Hardboiled Egg and a Granola Bar
Sweet Vanilla Smoothie – *RMD* – (1 cup)
Egg, hardboiled (1 egg)
Granola Bar [Quaker] (1 bar)

Morning Snack - 317 C / 310 S
Yogurt, Carrots and Graham Crackers
Yogurt, low fat (6 oz.)
Carrots (.5 cup)
Graham Crackers (2 large)

Lunch - 631 C / 586 S
Lentil Burger, Sunshine Pasta, Fruit Cocktail and Milk
Lentil Burger *RMD* (1 burger) on a whole-wheat bun (1 large) with romaine lettuce (1 leaf)
Sunshine Pasta Salad *RMD* (.5 cup)
Fruit cocktail, 1 cup
Milk, fat free (1 cup)

Afternoon Snack - 295 C / 560 S
Triscuits, Cheese and an Apple
Cheese [Laughing Cow] (2 wedges) on Triscuit whole-wheat crackers (6 crackers)
Apple (medium)

Dinner – 989 C / 478 S
Beef Mushroom Skillet with Broccoli, Rice, a Roll with Butter, and Banana Date Mousse
Beef Mushroom Skillet *RMD* (1 cup.)
Rice, brown (1 cup)
Broccoli, steamed (1 cup)
Roll, whole-wheat dinner (small)
Butter, unsalted (1t)
Banana Date Mousse *RMD* (.5 cup)

DASH Servings: .95 grain, 4.25 vegetables, 5.25 fruit, 4 dairy, 3 meat/fish/poultry, 0 nuts/ seeds

High Caloric - Day 5
Chicken Salad Sandwich / Beef Eye Round
2,503 C – 1,638 S

Breakfast - 673 C / 295 S
Granola Cereal with Toast and a Banana
Cereal, granola, oats, honey and almond [Quaker] (1 cup) with milk, fat free (1cup)
Bread, whole-wheat toasted (1 slice) with margarine (1t)
Banana (medium)

Morning Snack - 417 C / 100 S
Yogurt with Almonds and a Pear
Yogurt, low fat with fruit (6 oz.)
Almonds (.3 cup)
Pear (small)

Lunch - 436 C / 750 S
Chicken Salad Sandwich and Salad with Yogurt Dressing
Chicken salad - see recipe below (.8 cup)
Bread, whole-wheat (2 slices) with Dijon mustard (1t)
Iceberg lettuce (.3 cup); cucumber slices (.5 cup); carrot slices (.5 cup); and Yogurt
  Salad Dressing **RMD** (2T)

Afternoon Snack - 288 C / 147 S
Triscuit Crackers, Raisins and Fruit Cocktail
Triscuits, whole grain (6 crackers)
Raisins (.3 cup)
Fruit cocktail (.5 cup)

Dinner – 689 C / 346 S
Beef Eye Round with a Baked Potato, Sour Cream/Cheese and Green Beans
Beef Eye Round, lean, broiled or grilled (3 oz.)
Baked potato (small) with sour cream, low fat (2T) and cheddar cheese, low fat (1 0z.)
Green beans, cooked from frozen (1 cup)
Roll, whole-wheat (small) with margarine (1t)

DASH Servings: 8 grain, 6 vegetables, 4 fruit, 3.5 dairy, 5 meat/fish/poultry, 1 nuts/seeds

Chicken Salad Recipe (5 servings): 3 cups of cooked chicken breast diced, .25 cups of celery, 1 cup of sliced grapes, 1t of dill, .1t of salt, and 3T of mayonnaise, low fat.

High Caloric - Day 6
Shrimpy Spinach Salad / Stuffed Port Tenderloin
2,415 C – 2,431 S

Breakfast - 593 C / 685 S
Cereal, Bagel with Cream Cheese and a Banana
Cereal, TOTAL [General Mills] (1 cup); banana sliced (medium); milk, fat free (.5 cup)

Bagel, cinnamon-raisin (medium) with cream cheese, low fat (1T)

Morning Snack -331 C / 225 S
Canned Peaches with Almonds and String Cheese
Peaches, canned with light syrup (.5 cup)

Almonds (.3 cup)

String Cheese Lite, [Sargento] (2 pieces)

Lunch - 631 C / 459 S
Shrimpy Spinach Salad, White Bean Soup, Roll with Butter and Grape Juice
Shrimpy Spinach Salad with Asparagus **RMD** (1 cup)

White Bean Soup **RMD** (.75 cup)

Roll, whole wheat (small) with butter (1 tsp)

Grape juice (1 cup)

Afternoon Snack - 137 C / 82 S
Cantaloupe and Sourdough Pretzels
Cantaloupe (.5 cup)

Raisins (.3 cup)

Pretzels, unsalted sourdough [Snyder's] (20 mini)

Dinner – 723 C / 980 S
Stuffed Pork Tenderloin with Wild Rice, Carrots, a Roll, and a Vanilla Almond Parfait
Stuffed Pork Tenderloin **RMD** (3.5 oz.); Rice, wild (.5 cup)

Carrots (1 cup)

Roll, whole-wheat dinner (small) with butter (1tsp)

Vanilla Almond Parfait **RMD**, 1 cup

DASH Servings: 9.5 grain, 5 vegetables, 5.75 fruit, 2.8 dairy, 4.5 meat/fish/poultry, 1 nuts/seeds

High Caloric - Day 7
Veggy Mac and Cheese / Pasta Primavera
2,305 C – 2,055 S

Breakfast - 362 C / 519 S
Cheese Omelette with an English Muffin and Margarine, and an Apple
Egg substitute, [Eggbeaters] (.25 cup) with cheddar cheese (1 slice)
English muffin, cinnamon-raisin (medium) with margarine, soft (1t)
Apple (medium)

Morning Snack - 461 C / 337 S
Granola and Milk with Celery and Peanut Butter
Cereal, Granola [Open Nature] (.5 cup) with milk, fat free (1 cup)
Celery (1 7 inch stalk) with peanut butter (1T)

Lunch - 553 C / 276 S
Veggy Mac and Cheese, a Dinner Roll with Butter and Canned Peaches
Veggy Mac and Cheese *RMD* (1 cup)
Roll, standard dinner (small) with butter, unsalted (1tsp)
Peaches, canned (.5 cup)

Afternoon Snack - 376 C / 409 S
Tuna Salad with Triscuits and Grape Juice
Tuna, light in water (2 oz.); mayonnaise, reduced fat (1T); and celery, chopped (1T)
Triscuits, brown rice (6 Triscuits)
Grape juice (1 cup)

Dinner – 553 C / 514 S
Pasta Primavera, a Vinaigrette Salad, Dinner Roll with Margarine and Strawberry Jello
Pasta Primavera *RMD* (1.5 cups)
Lettuce, iceberg (1 cup) with cucumber slices (.3 cup) and Dijon Herb Vinaigrette Dressing *RMD* (2T)
Roll, whole-wheat (small) with margarine, soft (1t)
Jell-O [Spangles] (6 oz.)

DASH Servings: 7.5 grain, 4.25 vegetables, 5 fruit, 3 dairy, 2 meat/fish/poultry, 0.5 nuts/ seeds

Moderate Caloric Daily Meal Plans – 1,901 to 2,300 Calories

Moderate Caloric - Day 1
Split Pea Soup / Chicken and Dumplings
2,255 C – 2,069 S

Breakfast - 493 C / 320 S
Baked Banana, English Muffin with Margarine and Pineapple Juice
Baked Banana *RMD* (large)
English muffin, whole wheat (medium) with margarine, soft (1t)
Pineapple juice (1 cup)

Morning Snack - 299 C / 296 S
Triscuit Crackers with Cheese and an Apple
Triscuits, brown rice (6 Triscuits) with cheese, string [Sargento] (2 pcs)
Apple (medium)

Lunch - 484 C / 577 S
Split Pea Soup, Roll and Frozen Strawberry Yogurt
Split Pea Soup *RMD* (1 cup); with roll, whole wheat (small); and butter, unsalted (1t)
Yogurt, strawberry frozen [Yogurt-Land] (.5 cup)

Afternoon Snack - 324 C / 122 S
Butternut Cinnamon Smoothie and Cinnamon Sugar Pita Chips
Butternut Cinnamon Smoothie *RMD* (1 serving)
Pita chips, cinnamon sugar [Stacy's] (7 chips)

Dinner – 655 C / 754 S
Chicken and Dumplings, Roll with Butter and Coconut Sorbet
Chicken and Dumplings *RMD* (1 serving); with a roll, whole wheat (small); and butter
  (1t)
Milk, fat free (1 cup)
Coconut sorbet [Whole Fruit] (.5 cup)

DASH Servings: 8 grain, 4.5 vegetables, 6 fruit, 3 dairy, 2.5 meat/fish/poultry, 0 nuts/seeds

Moderate Caloric - Day 2
Grilled Mushroom Quesadilla / Filet Mignon
2,237 C – 2,032 S

Breakfast - 600 C / 673 S
Corn Flakes with Milk, Bagel with Cream Cheese and Peach Nectar
Cereal, corn flakes (2/3 cup) with milk, fat free (.5 cup)
Bagel, cinnamon-raisin (med) with cream cheese, low fat (2T)
Peach nectar (1 cup)

Morning Snack - 215 C / 0 S
Pineapple Slices with Almonds
Pineapple (2 slices)
Almonds (.3 cup)

Lunch - 674 C / 833 S
Grilled Mushroom Quesadilla with Sweet Potato Fries and an Apple
Grilled Mushroom Quesadilla **RMD** (1 serving) with sweet potato fries [Ore Ida] (3 oz.)
Apple (medium)

Afternoon Snack - 160 C / 285 S
Cheddar Cheese and Sourdough Pretzels
Cheese, lite cheddar [Laughing Cow](1 wedge)
Pretzels, sourdough [Snyder's] (20 mini)

Dinner – 588 C / 240 S
Filet Mignon and Mushrooms with a Baked Potato, Asparagus, a Dinner Roll and Peaches
Filet Mignon, barbequed or baked (3 oz.) with mushrooms, sliced (3 oz.)
Baked potato (medium) with butter, unsalted (1T)
Asparagus, cooked (.5 cup)
Roll, whole-wheat (small)
Peaches (.5 cup)

DASH Servings: 8 grain, 5.8 vegetables, 5.5 fruit, 3.6 dairy, 3 meat/fish/poultry, 1 nuts/seeds

Moderate Caloric - Day 3
Egg Salad Sandwich / Fish Tacos
2,144 C – 1,696 S

Breakfast - 344 C / 178 S
English Muffin with Butter and Jelly/Jam and Peaches
English muffin, cinnamon raisin (1 medium); butter, unsalted (1T); and jelly/jam
 [Smucker's] (1T)
Peaches, canned (.5 cup)

Morning Snack – 245 C / 66 S
Granola Bar with a Banana
Granola Bar, nut chewy [Quaker] (1 bar)
Banana (1 medium)

Lunch - 508 C / 555 S
**Egg Salad Sandwich with Lettuce on Rye Bread, Picnic Potato Salad, and
 Cantaloupe**
Egg, hard boiled and chopped (2 oz.), Mayonnaise, reduced fat (2T), celery, chopped
 (1T) on rye bread, 2 slices, with lettuce, romaine (1 leaf)
Baked French fries **RMD** (1 cup)
Cantaloupe (1 cup)

Afternoon Snack - 462 C / 428 S
Chex Mix Snack, Raisins and an Apple
Chex Mix, traditional snack mix (1 cup)
Raisins, (.3 cup)
Apple (1 medium)

Dinner – 585 C / 469 S
Fish Tacos with Steamed Broccoli
Halibut (2 X 3 oz. filet), tortilla (2 tortillas), avocado (2 oz.), lettuce, iceberg (.5 cup),
 and tartar sauce (2T)
Broccoli, steamed (.5 cup) with cheese, cheddar (1 oz.)

DASH Servings: 8 grain, 4.75 vegetables, 5.5 fruit, 2 dairy, 7 meat/fish/poultry, 1 nuts/seeds

Moderate Caloric - Day 4
Lentil Burger / Baked Halibut
2,142 C – 1,930 S

Breakfast - 541 C / 656 S
Bagel with Cream Cheese, Banana and Milk
Bagel, whole wheat (large) with cream cheese, low fat (2T)
Banana (medium)
Milk, fat free (1 cup)

Morning Snack - 369 C / 161 S
Fruit Yogurt with Sliced Carrots and Grape Juice
Yogurt, low fat with fruit (6 oz.)
Carrots, sliced (.5 cup)
Grape juice (1 cup)

Lunch - 352 C / 398 S
Lentil Burger with Cucumber Slices and an Apple
Lentil burger with whole-wheat bun *RMD* (1 burger)
Cucumber slices (6 oz.)
Apple (medium)

Afternoon Snack - 244 C / 389 S
Crackers with Hummus and Milk
Crackers, whole wheat (6) with hummus, roasted red pepper (2T)
Milk, fat free (1 cup)

Dinner – 636 C / 326 S
Baked Halibut, Baked Potato, Peas and Carrots, Roll and Jello
Baked halibut (4 oz.)
Potato, baked (.5 medium) with butter (1T)
Peas and carrots, (.5 cup)
Roll, whole-wheat dinner (small) with margarine (1t)
Jello, flavored (3.5 oz.)

DASH Servings: 7 grain, 5 vegetables, 5 fruit, 3 dairy, 5 meat/fish/poultry, 1 nuts/seeds

Moderate Caloric - Day 5
Turkey Burger / Gingersnap Beef Stew
2,127 C – 1,744 S

Breakfast - 554 C / 411 S
Raisin Bran with Milk, Toast with Margarine, Pineapple Juice and a Banana
Cereal, raisin bran (1 cup) with milk, fat free (.5 cup)
Bread, white toasted (2 slices) with margarine, soft (1t)
Pineapple juice (1 cup)

Morning Snack – 304 C / 104 S
Fruit Yogurt and Raisins
Yogurt, low fat with fruit (6 oz.)
Raisins (.3 cup)

Lunch - 492 C / 529 S
Turkey Burger on a Bun with Lettuce and Mayonnaise, Sweet Potato Fries, and Carrots
Turkey burger, [Jenny-O] (3 oz.) on a bun, whole wheat (1 regular); with mayonnaise, reduced fat, (1T); and romaine lettuce (1 leaf)
Sweet Potato Fries (3 oz.)
Carrot sticks (.5 cup)

Afternoon Snack - 338 C / 58 S
Apple Wheat Germ Smoothie and Almonds
Apple Wheat Germ Smoothie **RMD** (6 fl. oz.)
Almonds (.3 cup)

Dinner – 582 C / 729 S
Gingersnap Beef Stew, Spinach Salad, Steamed Broccoli, Cheddar Cheese, Roll and Butter
Gingersnap Beef Stew **RMD** (1 serving)
Spinach salad, instructions below 91cup)
Broccoli, steamed (1 cup)
Cheese, cheddar (1 oz.)
Roll, whole wheat (small) and butter (1t)

DASH Servings: 7.5 grain, 5.5 vegetables, 6 fruit, 3 dairy, 6 meat/fish/poultry, 1 nuts/seeds

Spinach Salad: 1 cup spinach leaves, ¼ cup grated carrots, and 2T vinaigrette dressing RMD

Moderate Caloric - Day 6
Tuna Melt / Curry Almond Chicken
1,983 C – 2,050 S

Breakfast - 350 C / 399 S
Quiche with Asparagus, Milk and a Banana
Quiche with Asparagus **RMD** (1 slice)
Milk, fat free (.5 cup)
Banana (1 medium)

Morning Snack – 385 C / 423 S
Yogurt with Fruit, English Muffin with Margarine and Carrots
Yogurt, low fat with fruit (6 oz.)
English muffin, whole wheat (1 medium) with margarine, soft (2t)
Carrots (.5 cup)

Lunch - 410 C / 713 S
Tuna Melt Sandwich with Grape Juice
Tuna, light in water (2 oz.); bread, whole wheat (2 slices); cheese, cheddar (1 oz.);
  celery, chopped (1T); and mayonnaise, reduced fat (1T)
Grape juice (.5 cup)

Afternoon Snack - 306 C / 152 S
Crackers, Raisins and an Apple
Crackers, whole wheat (6 crackers)
Raisins (.3 cup)
Apple (1 medium)

Dinner –532 C / 363 S
Baked Chicken and Rice, Green Beans, Roll with Margarine and Fruit Cocktail
Baked Chicken and Rice **RMD** (1 serving)
Green beans from frozen (1 cup)
Roll, whole-wheat dinner (1 small) with margarine, soft (1t)
Fruit cocktail (.5 cup)

DASH Servings: 6.5 grain, 4.75 vegetables, 5 fruit, 3.5 dairy, 5.25 meat/fish/poultry, 0 nuts/ seeds

Moderate Caloric - Day 7
Chicken Sandwich / Tuna Casserole
1,927 C – 2,313 S

Breakfast - 395 C / 459 S
Cheese and Mushroom Omelet, Sweet Pea Smoothie, and Bread with Butter
Egg substitute [Eggbeaters] (.5 cup); with mushrooms, sliced, fresh (1 oz.); cheese, cheddar (.5 oz.)
Sweet Pea Smoothie **RMD** (1 cup)
Bread, whole wheat (1 slice) with butter, unsalted (1t)

Morning Snack – 247 C / 120 S
Yogurt with Pineapple and a Pear
Yogurt, low fat, plain (6 oz.) with pineapple pieces (2 slices)
Pear (1 small)

Lunch - 585 C / 607 S
Chicken Sandwich with Mayonnaise and Lettuce, Sweet Potato Fries, Cucumbers and an Apple
Chicken breast, cooked (2 oz.) on bread, whole wheat (2 slices) with mayonnaise, low fat (1T) and lettuce, romaine (1 leaf)
Sweet Potato Fries (3 oz.)
Cucumbers, sliced (.5 cup)
Apple (1 medium)

Afternoon Snack - 165 C / 253 S
Crackers with Cheese and Peaches
Crackers, whole wheat, low salt (6 crackers) with cheese, cheddar (1 oz.)
Peaches, canned (.5 cup)

Dinner – 535 C / 674 S
Tuna Casserole, Corn, Roll with margarine, and Frozen Yogurt
Tuna casserole RMD (1 cup)
Corn, sweet, yellow, canned (.5 cup)
Roll, whole wheat (1 small) with margarine, soft (1t)
Yogurt, frozen, vanilla, low fat Greek [Yoplait] (.5 cup)

DASH Servings: 7 grain, 4.75 vegetables, 5 fruit, 3 dairy, 4 meat/fish/poultry, 0 nuts/seeds

Low Caloric Daily Meal Plans – 1,600 to 1,900 Calories

Low Caloric - Day 1
Chicken Pita / Fish in Parchment
1,862 C – 1,660 S

Breakfast - 295 C / 286 S
Cheerios with Milk and Bananas
Cereal, Cheerios (1 cup) with milk, fat free (1 cup), and a banana (medium)

Morning Snack - 479 C / 75 S
Yogurt with Strawberry Jelly, Almonds and Raisins
Yogurt, fat free [Chobani] (5,3 oz.) with jam, strawberry [Smucker's] (2T)
Almonds (.3 cup) and raisins (.3 cup)

Lunch - 451 C / 590 S
Chicken Pita with a Pear
Chicken, broiled (3 oz.); pita bread (regular); cucumbers, sliced (.5 cups); carrots,
   shredded (.3 cup); lettuce, iceberg, shredded (.3 cup); and ranch dressing, fat free (1T)
Pear (small)

Afternoon Snack - 147 C / 171 S
Bagel with Cream Cheese and Grapes
Bagel, (mini) with cream cheese, low fat (1T)
Grapes, red or green (.5 cup)

Dinner – 490C / 538 S
Fish Filet in Parchment, Broccoli with Cheese, Roll with Butter and Jell-O
Fish Filet in Parchment *RMD* (4.0z.)
Broccoli, steamed (.5 cup) with cheese, cheddar low fat (1 oz.)
Roll, whole wheat (small) with butter (1t)
Jell-O [Spangles] (6 oz.)

DASH Servings: 5 grain, 5 vegetables, 4.5 fruit, 2.8 dairy, 7 meat/fish/poultry, 0 nuts/seeds

Low Caloric - Day 2
Cobb Salad / Braised Short Ribs

1,839 C – 2,193 S

Breakfast - 534 C / 289 S
Fruit Yogurt, English Muffin with Jelly, and Grape Juice

Yogurt, fat free with fruit (.5 cup)

English muffin, cinnamon-raisin (medium) with jelly or jam [Smucker's] (1T)

Grape juice (1 cup)

Morning Snack - 427 C / 175 S
Celery with Peanut Butter, Almonds and an Apple

Celery (7-inch stalk) with peanut butter (2T)

Almonds (.3cup)

Apple (medium)

Lunch - 215 C / 742 S
Cobb Salad with a Roll and Butter

Lettuce, iceberg (1 cup); ham, 11% fat, chopped (1 slice); turkey, chopped [Columbus]
(1 slice); celery, chopped (5 inch stalk); and yogurt dressing **RMD** (2T)

Roll, whole wheat (small) with butter (1t)

Afternoon Snack - 202 C / 357 S
Cheese and Crackers with Apple Juice

Cracker, whole wheat (6 crackers) with cheese, cheddar low fat (2 oz.)

Apple juice (.5 cup)

Dinner – 461C / 630S
Braised Short Ribs, Rice, Spinach, Roll with Margarine, and Pineapple Juice

Braised short ribs **RMD** (2 ribs)

Rice, long grain brown (.5 cup)

Spinach, cooked from frozen (.5 cup)

Roll, whole wheat (small) with margarine (1t)

Pineapple juice (.5 cup)

DASH Servings: 6 grain, 4.75 vegetables, 5 fruit, 2.5 dairy, 5 meat/fish/poultry, 2 nuts/seeds

Low Caloric - Day 3
Chicken Quesadilla / Mustard Pork Loin
1,829 C – 2,189 S

Breakfast - 558 C / 588 S
Sweet Pea Smoothie, Bagel with Cream Cheese and Milk
Sweet Pea Smoothie *RMD* (1 cup)
Bagel, whole wheat (large) with cream cheese, low fat (1 T)
Milk, fat free (.5 cup)

Morning Snack - 157 C / 465 S
Cottage Cheese with Fruit Cocktail
Cottage cheese, 2% (.5 cup)
Fruit cocktail (.5 cup)

Lunch - 238 C / 287 S
Chicken Quesadilla, Spinach Salad with Yogurt Dressing and Cucumber Slices
Corn tortilla (1 standard); cheese, Colby low fat (1 oz.); chicken breast, cooked (2 oz.);
   margarine, soft (1 t)
Spinach (1 cup) with yogurt dressing RMD (2 T)
Cucumbers, sliced (.5 cup)

Afternoon Snack - 314 C / 164 S
Granola Bar with Fruit Yogurt
Granola Bar, Nut Chew [Quaker] (1 bar)
Yogurt, low fat with fruit (6 oz.)

Dinner – 562 C / 686 S
Mustard Pork Loin with Long Grain Rice, Broccoli, Roll with Margarine and Peach
   Nectar
Mustard Pork Loin *RMD* (4 oz.)
Rice, long grain, brown (.5 up)
Broccoli, steamed (1 cup)
Roll, whole wheat (1 small) with Margarine (1 t)
Peach nectar (.5 cup)

DASH Servings: 5 grain, 4 vegetables, 4 fruit, 3.5 dairy, 6 meat/fish/poultry, 0.5 nuts/seeds

Low Caloric - Day 4
Chicken Salad / Oven Steamed Tilapia
1,837 C – 1,402 S

Breakfast - 406 C / 272 S
Instant Oatmeal, English Muffin with Margarine, a Banana and Milk
Instant Oatmeal, regular (.5 cup)
English muffin, cinnamon-raisin (medium) with margarine, soft, (1t)
Milk, fat free (.5 cup)

Morning Snack - 425 C / 102 S
Fruit Yogurt with an Apple and Almonds
Yogurt, low fate with fruit (6 oz.)
Apple (medium)
Almonds (.3 cup)

Lunch - 262 C / 246 S
Chicken Salad on a Bed of Lettuce, Cucumbers, and Sourdough Pretzels
Chicken Salad – see recipe below (.8 cup) on lettuce, iceberg (1 cup)
Cucumber, sliced (.5 cup)
Pretzels, sourdough, unsalted [Snyder's] (10 mini)

Afternoon Snack - 307 C / 358 S
String Cheese on Triscuits with a Pear
Cheese, string, lite [Sargento] (2 pieces) on Triscuit crackers, whole grain (6 crackers)
Pear (small)

Dinner – 437 C / 404 S
Oven Steamed Tilapia with Rice, Spinach Salad, Roll with Butter and Cheddar Cheese
Oven steamed tilapia **RMD**, steamed (4 oz.) with rice, wild (.5 cup)
Spinach (1 cup); cucumbers, sliced (.25 cup); carrots, shredded (.25 cup); and Vinaigrette dressing **RMD** (2T)
Roll, whole wheat (1 small) with butter (1t)
Cheese, cheddar low fat (1 oz.)

DASH Servings: 7 grain, 4 vegetables, 3.5 fruit, 3.5 dairy, 6 meat/fish/poultry, 1 nuts/seeds

Chicken Salad Recipe (5 servings): 3 cups of cooked chicken breast diced, .25 cups of celery, 1 cup of sliced grapes, 1t of dill, .1t of salt, and 3T of mayonnaise, low fat.

Low Caloric - Day 5
Grilled Cheese / Shrimp and Pea Stir Fry
1,769 C – 2,117 S

Breakfast - 254 C / 72 S
Frost Wheat Cereal with Milk and Fruit Cocktail
Cereal, frosted wheat [Fiber One] (.5 cup) with milk, fat free (.5 cup)
Fruit cocktail (1 cup)

Morning Snack - 301 C / 197 S
Apple Wheat Germ Smoothie with a Bagel and Jelly or Jam
Apple Wheat Germ Smoothie *RMD* (1 cup)
Bagel (mini) with jelly or jam [Smucker's] (1T)

Lunch - 441 C / 908 S
Grilled Turkey and Cheese Sandwich with Carrots
Bread, whole wheat [Safeway] (2 slices); cheese, provolone, low fat (1 slice); turkey, low
  sodium [Columbus] (2 slices); and margarine (1T)
Carrots, sliced (.5 cup)

Afternoon Snack - 213 C / 519 S
Cucumber Salad and Crackers with Hummus
Cucumber Salad *RMD* (.5 cup)
Crackers, wheat thins [Nabisco] (10 crackers) with Hummus, Greek olive [Sabra] (2T

Dinner – 560 C / 421 S
**Shrimp and Pea Stir Fry, Roll with Margarine, Milk, and Strawberry Cream with
  Mango**
Shrimp and Pea Stir Fry *RMD* (1.3 cup)
Roll, whole wheat (1 small) with margarine (1t)
Strawberry Cream with Mango *RMD* (1 cup)
Milk, fat free (1 cup)

DASH Servings: 6 grain, 4 vegetables, 4.5 fruit, 3 dairy, 4 meat/fish/poultry, 1 nuts/seeds

Low Caloric - Day 6
Vegetable and White Bean Soup / Roasted Salmon
1,715 C – 1,686 S

Breakfast - 290 C / 125 S
Frosted Shredded Wheat with Milk
Frosted Shredded Wheat [Fiber One] (1 cup) with milk, fat free (1 cup)

Morning Snack - 298 C / 254 S
Yogurt with Raisins, Toast with Margarine
Yogurt, fat free [Chobani] (5,3 oz.) with raisins (1 oz.)
Bread, whole wheat, toasted, [Safeway] (1 slice) with margarine, soft (1t)

Lunch - 299 C / 355 S
Vegetable and White Bean Soup with a Roll and Margarine and an Apple
Vegetable and White Bean Soup **RMD** (.8 cup)
Roll, whole wheat (small) with margarine (1t)
Apple (medium)

Afternoon Snack - 302 C / 250 S
Bagel with Jelly, Cantaloupe, and Cashews
Bagel, whole wheat (.5 medium) with jelly [Smucker's] (1T)
Cashews, dry roasted, no salt added (1T)
Cantaloupe (1 cup)

Dinner – 526C / 702S
Salmon with Mango Honey Glaze, Rice, and Broccoli with Cheese
Salmon with Mango Honey **RMD** (6 oz. filet)
Rice, long grain brown (.5 cup)
Broccoli, steamed (1 cup) with cheese, cheddar low fat (2 oz.)

DASH Servings: 6 grain, 4 vegetables, 4 fruit, 3.5 dairy, 6 meat/fish/poultry, .5 nuts/seeds

Low Caloric - Day 7
Shrimp Pita / Vegetable Chowder
1,638 C – 1,799 S

Breakfast - 273 C / 491 S
Egg and English Muffin with Milk
Egg substitute [Eggbeaters] (,25 cup); English muffin, whole wheat (medium); and
   margarine, soft (1t)
Milk, fat free (1 cup)

Morning Snack - 302 C / 176 S
Butternut Squash Smoothie with Graham Crackers
Butternut Squash Smoothie **RMD** (1 cup)
Graham crackers (2 large)

Lunch - 394 C / 550 S
Shrimp Pita and an Apple
Shrimp, cooked (3 oz.); pita bread, whole wheat (regular); cucumbers, sliced (.5 cups);
   lettuce, iceberg, shredded (.3 cup); and tartar sauce (1t)
Apple (large)

Afternoon Snack - 162 C / 356 S
Cheese and Turkey on Triscuit Melt
Triscuits, whole grain (6 Triscuits); with cheese, cheddar low fat (1 oz.); and turkey, low
   sodium [Columbus] (1 oz.)

Dinner – 507 C / 226 S
Vegetable Chowder with a Spinach Salad and Strawberry Creams
Vegetable Chowder **RMD** (1 cup)
Spinach (1 cup) with raisins (.3 cup) and Vinaigrette dressing **RMD** *(2T)*
Strawberry Creams **RMD** (1 serving)

DASH Servings: 6 grain, 4.5 vegetables, 4.5 fruit, 2 dairy, 4 meat/fish/poultry, 0 nuts/seeds

Section VI
Recipes

Recipe Index

Main courses

Grilled mushroom quesadilla

Pasta primavera with whole wheat pasta

"Guilt-free" chicken and dumplings

California fried chicken

Baked chicken and wild rice

Healthy pot pie

Enchiladas verde

Chicken and mushroom cheese bake

Curry almond chicken

Slow cooker Sunday supper

Stuffed turkey rolls "Cordon Bleu"

Turkey stroganoff

Whole wheat empanadas

Mustard pork loin with cauliflower puree

Stuffed pork tenderloin

Easy beef (or pork) burgundy

Gingersnap beef stew with red cabbage

Beef and mushroom skillet

Braised short ribs

Oven steamed tilapia

Shrimp and pea stir fry

Roasted salmon with mango honey soy glaze

Elegant dover sole

Fish fillets in parchment

Grilled Caesar swordfish

White fish Veronica

Trout almondine

Tuna casserole

Sides

Healthy cornbread

Homestyle southern biscuits

Savory Italian vegetables

Sweet potato custard

Twice baked potatoes

Carolina potato pie

Baked French fries

Risotto with parsley and seasonal vegetables

Ginger pasta pilaf

Exotic Asian rice

Vegetable macaroni and cheese

Mini lasagna cups

Stuffed mushroom caps

Treats

Cantaloupe sorbet

Pineapple ambrosia

Vanilla almond parfait

Baked bananas

Peachy cobbler

Banana date mousse

Coconut rice pudding

Strawberry cream with mango and honey sauce

Peanut butter milkshake

Oats, nuts, and berry breakfast

Breakfast is the most important meal of the day, so we think it should be hearty and healthy. This baked recipe contains nutritious oats, chia seeds, chopped almonds, berries, and quinoa. If you are not familiar with quinoa (pronounced "keen wa") it is considered a superfood grain because of its powerful health benefits. High in protein, fiber, and amino acids, quinoa is also flavorful and tasty enough when cooked to be used in all sorts of foods these days. This GERD diet friendly breakfast recipe is surprisingly filling, and will surely keep those mid-morning hunger pangs at bay! It's multi-textured and so delicious!

Yields about 6 servings

Ingredients

2-3/4 cups low-fat milk
1/4 cup melted butter
1 TBSP vanilla extract
1 cup old fashioned oats
1/2 cup chopped almonds
3/4 cup quinoa
1/2 cup brown sugar
2 TBSP chia seeds
1 tsp baking powder
1/4 tsp salt
1 cup blueberries
2 cups chopped strawberries

Directions

1. Preheat oven to 375 degrees.
2. Spray 2 quart baking dish with nonstick cooking spray.
3. In medium bowl, whisk together the 2 3/4 cups low-fat milk, 1/4 cup melted butter, and 1 TBSP vanilla.
4. Place oats in the baking dish and add quinoa, roasted almonds, brown sugar, chia seeds, baking powder, and salt.
5. Pour milk mixture over the ingredients and top with berries.
6. Bake for about 50 minutes or until liquid is absorbed.

Nutritional information (per serving): Calories 455, Sodium 380mg

'Design your own' breakfast granola

Granola is very expensive to buy at the store, but very inexpensive to make at home, so put on your creative hat and give this recipe a try. It's easy because granola is basically just rolled oats to which you can add your choice of dried fruits, nuts, and other tasty tidbits. You can also tweak the mixture with GERD diet friendly spices like cinnamon and ginger. Add the spices and ingredients like brown sugar, grated apple and coconut before baking. Other choices like dried fruits, nuts, and raisins should be added after baking. It's a pretty forgiving recipe, so feel free to have fun while customizing your own blend!

Ingredients

6 cups rolled oats
6 cups wheat germ
1 cup salad oil
1 cup honey
Plus your favorite extras like spices, coconut, raisins, almonds, or other nuts and dried fruits

Directions

1. Mix oats and wheat germ in large bowl.
2. Mix oil and honey together, then add to the first mixture.
3. If you're using extra ingredients like spices, brown sugar, grated apple, or coconut, add them before baking.
4. Bake at 350 degrees on cookie sheets for 15 minutes.
5. You may need to stir with a fork to make sure all gets dry.
6. Add your extras like raisins, almonds, other nuts or dried fruit and stir.
7. Let set to cool, then store in an airtight container.

Nutritional information (per half cup serving): Approximately 120 calories, Sodium 31mg, but this is largely dependent on what you add. When customizing your own blend, use the "food search" at www.calorieking.com and type in your choice of ingredients to determine the values for your granola.

Homemade granola parfait

This versatile recipe has it all: protein, fiber, healthy fats, and lots of vitamins and minerals. Try it today for breakfast or a healthy snack! This recipe is great for a quick, healthy breakfast because it's loaded with nutrition: fiber from the oats, protein from the Greek yogurt, healthy fats from the almonds, and vitamins and minerals from the fruit. It also perfect to bring to a brunch and can make a nice gift. Healthy and delicious!

Recipes serves 16 (1/4 cup per serving)

Ingredients

For Granola	*For Parfait*
4 cups dry steel cut oats	¼ cup granola
½ cup sliced almonds	*1 cup Greek nonfat yogurt*
¼ cup brown sugar	½ cup Seasonal berries
½ tsp salt	
½ tsp cinnamon	
¼ cup canola oil	
¼ cup honey	
1 tsp vanilla	
¼ currant	

Directions
1. Preheat oven to 300 degrees.
2. In a large bowl mix the oats, almonds, brown sugar, salt, and cinnamon.
3. In a saucepan heat the oil and honey and whisk in the vanilla.
4. Once warm, pour the oil and honey mixture over the oats in the bowl and stir to coat the dry ingredients with the wet mixture.
5. Spread the granola on a large cookie sheet.
6. Bake at 300 degrees for 40 minutes, removing to stir every 10 minutes.
7. Let cool completely and then store in an airtight container.
8. To make a parfait, place the yogurt in a bowl and top with berries and granola.

Nutritional Information Granola (per serving): Calories 200, Sodium 74mg

Nutritional Information Parfait (per serving): Calories 354, Sodium 160mg

Good morning fruit salad

A fruit salad is a nice and healthy way to start your day. This recipe is made with GERD-friendly fruits including kiwi, which adds a tropical flair to the dish. Kiwifruits are rich in fiber and contain as much vitamin C as an orange, a citrus fruit most people with acid reflux avoid. When selecting kiwifruits, make sure they yield gently to pressure and avoid those that are very soft or bruised. The slicing and peeling for this mixture will take a little effort, but it will last at least a few days in the refrigerator, so give it a try!

Ingredients

For fruit salad

2 golden delicious apples, peeled and chopped

1 pint strawberries, sliced

3 kiwi fruits, peeled, seeded and chopped*

1 cantaloupe, peeled, seeded and chopped

1/2 tsp apple cider vinegar

2 TBSP slivered almonds

For vanilla Greek yogurt sauce

8 TBSP vanilla Greek Yogurt

2 TBSP Apple Cider vinegar

2 TBSP Honey

Directions

1. Place apples in a large bowl and toss with 1/2 tsp apple cider vinegar.
2. Add all remaining ingredients, except kiwi, and mix well.
3. To prepare the yogurt sauce, mix the yogurt with the vinegar and honey in a small bowl. Whisk well and store in the refrigerator until ready to serve.
4. When ready to serve, add the kiwifruits to each bowl, and top each serving with desired amount of yogurt sauce.

*Kiwifruit should be added last minute to the salad because it will make the other fruit overly soft. Any kiwi "leftovers" should be stored in a separate container.

Nutritional Information (per one cup serving of fruit): Calories 116, Sodium 2mg

Nutritional information (for 1 TBSP of yogurt sauce): Calories 12, Sodium 5mg

Creamy zucchini quiche

With plenty of veggies and a creamy reduced-fat egg and cheese filling, this light and fluffy quiche is ideal for breakfast or brunch. For these warm wedges, we used fresh zucchini, red bell pepper, and celery seasoned up Italian style, but this quiche recipe is versatile, and you can easily make substitutions of similar amounts of GERD diet friendly veggies and spices. It's quick to prepare and freezes well too. The dish is almost a meal in itself, so all you will need is a green salad or some fresh fruit on the side. It's family pleasing and so delicious!

Yields about 8 servings

Ingredients

1 unbaked 9-inch piecrust
4 cups grated zucchini
1/2 cup finely chopped red pepper
1/2 cup finely chopped celery
1 tsp oregano
1/2 tsp dried basil
1 tsp dried parsley
2 eggs (or appropriate amount of egg substitute)
1/2 cup fat-free half and half
3/4 cup shredded reduced-fat mozzarella cheese
3/4 reduced-fat sharp cheddar cheese

Directions

1. Preheat oven to 375 degrees.
2. Press piecrust into deep dish pie plate and flute the edges.
3. Sauté vegetables for about 4 minutes until tender in a large skillet sprayed with nonstick cooking spray. Remove from heat and stir in oregano, basil, and parsley flakes.
4. Whisk eggs well in a large bowl and stir in half and half. Add the cheese and mix well. Fold in vegetables, and slowly pour the mixture into the prepared pie plate.
5. Bake about 30 to 35 minutes. The quiche is done when a knife inserted in the center of the quiche comes out clean.
6. Cover with foil and let stand for 15 to 20 minutes to ensure that the quiche will not fall apart.

Nutritional information (per serving): About 200 calories, Sodium 390mg

Asparagus Quiche

Who doesn't love going out to breakfast and ordering the healthy veggie quiche? But who knew what you are eating actually is full of cream butter and cheese? That's a lot of dairy and a lot of regret later. We created this great recipe for a great tasting healthy quiche that fills you up with protein instead of fat. It tastes and looks like you put a lot of work into it, but it's really quite simple.

We did a few things make this traditional recipe healthier. Turkey bacon replaces regular bacon to reduce the fat. Swiss and Parmesan cheeses are used, which are full of flavor, allowing you to use less and reduce the overall fat content of the recipe, but still get the satisfaction of cheese. BUT the main culprit in this dish is cream; half and half, which is the lowest fat cream, still contains 18% fat! Replacing the cream it with plain, nonfat yogurt creates the same creamy texture, but is so much better for your health.

Recipe serves 8

Ingredients

1 unbaked, 9-inch piecrust
½ pound asparagus cut into ¼ inch pieces (or between 1 and 1 ½ cups)
6 turkey bacon strips, cooked to desired crispness and chopped
2 TBSP green onion or chives
3 eggs (or 2 eggs and 2 egg whites/ 1 egg and 3 egg whites)
1 ½ cups nonfat or low- fat plain yogurt (Greek yogurt can be used but may be more tart in flavor)
½ cups Swiss cheese
¼ cups Parmesan cheese
½ tsp salt
1/8 tsp nutmeg

Directions

1. Preheat the oven to 450 degrees, cover piecrust with aluminum foil and bake for 5 minutes, remove the foil, and bake for 5 additional minutes.
2. Steam asparagus until bright green and tender, but still crisp (approximately 4-5 minutes).
3. While the asparagus is cooking, beat the eggs in a bowl and slowly add the yogurt ½ cup at a time.
4. Add in the nutmeg, salt, chives and stir.
5. Slowly add in the cheeses, leaving a small amount to sprinkle on the top of the quiche.
6. Once bacon is cooked, add to the egg mixture.

7. When the piecrust is finished and the asparagus has been steamed, spread the asparagus across the bottom of the piecrust.
8. Slowly pour the egg-yogurt mixture over the top of the asparagus; this will give the final product a layered look.
9. Sprinkle the remaining cheese on top of the quiche.
10. Reduce the oven temperature to 400 degrees and bake the quiche in for 10 minutes, then reduce the heat 350 degrees and continue baking for 25-30 minutes. The quiche is done when a knife is inserted in the center of the quiche and come out clean.
11. Let stand 15-20 minutes before serving. This ensures the quiche will not fall apart.

Nutritional information (per serving): Calories 200, Sodium 335mg

Whole Wheat Banana Walnut Scones

Smart modifications turn this sweet indulgence into a breakfast with plenty of fiber and healthy fat. These scones have half the fat of traditional scones, but include plenty of good fats with the addition of flaxseeds and walnuts. This recipe works well for people with GERD because the scones are very filling, but low fat and low in calories. The scones also freeze well, so double the recipe and freeze the leftovers. Just reheat them in the microwave for 30 seconds and they still taste great!

Recipe serves 8

Ingredients

1 ¼ cups oatmeal
1 ¼ cups whole wheat flour
¼ cup brown sugar
2 TBSP ground flax seeds
1 tsp baking powder
½ tsp baking soda
½ cup smart balance
⅔ cup plain non-fat yogurt
1 mashed banana
¼ cup walnut pieces
¼ cup mini chocolate chips (*if desired or tolerable*)

Directions

1. Whisk together oatmeal, flour, sugar, baking powder, soda, flax seeds.
2. Add Smart Balance and "cut in" or blend with a pastry blender or fork. The mixture should look like coarse crumbs.
3. Add the yogurt and banana and stir until mixture sticks together.
4. Stir in walnuts and chocolate chips.
5. Either scoop mixture with an ice cream scoop (to make it easy) or make the scone mixture into a circle and cut like a pizza and this will make 8 scones.
6. Place scones on a parchment paper lined cookie sheet (wax paper works, too).
7. Stack two cookies sheets to prevent the bottoms from burning. Bake at 400 degrees for 15-20 minutes.

Nutritional information (per serving): Calories 196, Sodium 100mg

Apple pecan coffee cake

Apples and raisins provide the moistness for this yummy coffee cake recipe, so we were able to use less oil to keep it low in saturated fat and GERD diet friendly. We add vanilla for flavor, chopped pecans for crunch, and cinnamon for seasoning. This yummy cake is perfect with your morning coffee or is a delicious treat any time of day! The mixture will fill your 9 x 13 pan to the brim, so be sure you have someone to enjoy it with!

Recipe serves 20

Ingredients

5 cups tart apples, cored, peeled, and chopped
1 cup sugar
1 cup dark raisins
1/2 cup pecans, chopped
1/4 cup vegetable oil
2 tsp vanilla
1 egg beaten
2-1/2 cup sifted all-purpose flour
1-1/2 tsp baking soda
2 tsp ground cinnamon

Directions

1. Preheat oven to 350 degrees F.
2. Lightly oil a 13x9x2-inch pan.
3. In a large mixing bowl, combine apples with sugar, raisins, and pecans; mix well. Let stand 30 minutes.
4. Stir in oil, vanilla, and egg. Sift together flour, baking soda, and cinnamon.
5. Stir into apple mixture about 1/3 at a time just enough to moisten dry ingredients.
6. Turn batter into pan. Bake 35 to 40 minutes. Cool cake slightly before serving.

Nutritional information (per serving): 188 Calories, Sodium 68mg

Raisin pecan and carrot bread

This tasty bread recipe is low in saturated fat and is made with carrots, raisins, and pecans, all acid reflux friendly ingredients. We use a small amount of egg in the recipe, but an egg substitute will also work well for those who need to minimize eggs in their GERD diet plan. I make this often because my family loves it! It's easy, healthy, and so enjoyable!

Recipe makes one loaf (Serving size 1/2 inch slice)

Ingredients

1-1/2 sifted all-purpose flour
1/2 cup sugar
1 tsp baking powder
1/4 tsp baking soda
1/2 tsp salt
1-1/2 tsp ground cinnamon
1/4 tsp ground allspice
1 egg, beaten
1/2 cup water
2 TBSP vegetable oil
1/2 tsp vanilla
1-1/2 finely shredded carrots
1/4 cup chopped pecans
1/4 cup golden raisins

Directions

1. Preheat oven to 350 degrees.
2. Lightly oil a 9 x 5 x 3 inch loaf pan.
3. Stir together dry ingredients in large mixing bowl and make a well in the center of dry mixture.
4. In separate bowl, mix together remaining ingredients. Add this mixture all at once to dry ingredients. Stir just enough to moisten and evenly distribute carrots.
5. Turn into prepared pan. Bake for 50 minutes or until toothpick inserted in center comes out clean.
6. Cool 5 minutes in pan. Remove from pan and complete cooling on a wire rack before slicing.

Nutritional information: Calories 99, Sodium 12mg

Butternut squash and cinnamon smoothie

Lightly cooked butternut squash makes this an unusual, but delicious, vitamin packed smoothie. Squash has a wonderful rich flavor that's enhanced by the addition of apples, peaches, and cinnamon for this GERD diet friendly recipe. This feel good drink is quite luxurious, and works best as a lunchtime meal substitution! Give it a try! It's an energizing blend and a sweet superfood treat!

Yields two servings

Ingredients

1 small butternut squash (6 oz)
1/2 tsp ground cinnamon
1 cup apple juice
1 cup peach juice

Directions

1. Halve the squash, and scoop out and discard seeds.
2. Peel the squash and cut into chunks.
3. Steam the squash 10 minutes or until tender.
4. Drain well and cool.
5. Put squash in blender.
6. Add cinnamon and juices.
7. Process ingredients until smooth.
8. Add a few ice cubes to two small glasses and serve immediately.

Nutritional information (per serving): Calories 184, Sodium 7mg

Tasty tofu smoothie

This creative recipe is bursting with goodness, and just what you need to get your morning off to a great start! Why tofu? Because tofu is not only rich in minerals, it's also a perfect natural source of protein. Drink this creamy blend with cereal or a slice of toast, and it should easily see you through until lunchtime. This "superfood" treat is GERD diet friendly so give it a try, and experience the sweet flavors!

Recipe makes 2 servings

Ingredients

9 oz firm tofu
2 cups strawberries
3 TBSP sunflower seeds
1 1/2 cups mango or guava juice
1/4 tsp sunflower seed for topping

Directions

1. Coarsely chop tofu.
2. Chop strawberries (remove hulls), and reserve a few chunks.
3. Put all ingredients in a blender or food processor, and blend until smooth.
4. Pour the smoothie into glasses.
5. Top with remaining sunflower seeds and strawberry chunks.

Nutritional information (per serving): Calories 268, Sodium 18mg

Apple wheat germ smoothie

This is a GERD diet friendly, carbohydrate-rich, concoction that is sure to give you an invigorating boost! It makes a nice mid-morning or afternoon snack. Wheat germ is the most nutritious part of the wheat grain. It's packed with protein, minerals and vitamins B and E, making it a super healthy addition to any smoothie. Pour it into your blender, add yogurt, a ripe banana, apple juice, a tablespoon of flax seeds, and voila! This recipe makes a perfect tonic for general well being in just seconds!

Makes two 6 oz. servings

Ingredients

2 TBSP wheat germ
1 large ripe banana
1/2 cup plain yogurt
1 TBSP flax seeds
1 cup apple juice
1/4 cup water

Directions

1. Place the wheat germ, 2/3 of the banana, yogurt and flax seeds in a blender or food processor.
2. Blend until smooth and stir well.
3. Add the apple juice to the mixture and blend again.
4. Pour into a large glass and top with water and remaining banana slices.

Nutritional information (per serving): Calories 179, Sodium 58mg

Icy mango smoothie

Mangoes taste so good that people might forget that they are also healthy, containing high amounts of fiber, iron, and antioxidants. Its fruit flavor is often described as an exotic mix of pineapple and peach. Sounds delicious! And on top of that, they are GERD diet friendly and do not promote heartburn symptoms. Adults and children alike will love the creamy sweet taste of this drink! It's a perfect breakfast for your GERD diet plan or any time of day as a meal substitution.

Makes 4 servings (3/4 cup per serving)

Ingredients
2 cups 1% milk
4 TBSP frozen mango juice or 1 fresh pitted mango*
1 small banana
1/4 tsp ginger
2 ice cubes

Directions
1. Put all ingredients into a blender.
2. Blend until foamy. Serve immediately.

*When choosing a ripe mango for this recipe, stay away from very soft or bruised fruit. A fresh mango will give slightly to the touch and will have a tropical fruit aroma.

Nutritional information (per serving): Calories 106, Sodium 63mg

Sweet vanilla smoothie

We like to try a variety of smoothies during the week to add extra servings of fruits and vegetables to our GERD friendly diet. This recipe uses a ripe banana, pineapple and strawberries, which are non-acidic fruits that should not trigger your acid reflux symptoms. The dash of vanilla perks up the nonfat yogurt and gives this smoothie just the right flavor. So sweet!

Makes 3 one cup servings

Ingredients

1 cup yogurt, plain nonfat
6 medium strawberries
1 cup pineapple, crushed, canned in juice
1 medium ripe banana
1 tsp vanilla extract
4 ice cubes

Directions

1. Place all ingredients in a blender and purée until smooth.
2. Serve in a chilled glass.

Nutritional information (per serving): Calories 121, Sodium 64mg

Carrot milkshake smoothie

This smoothie recipe is a perfect quick and healthy breakfast for an "on the go" morning. If you like carrot cake, you will enjoy the milkshake texture of this smoothie, and the combination of carrots, milk, banana, and cinnamon make it mmm mmm delicious! This heartburn friendly treat is also a great way to satisfy your sweet tooth any time of the day, while adding some extra fruit and veggies to your acid reflux friendly diet.

Ingredients

1 large firm carrot
4 or 5 spinach leaves
*1 cup of low-fat (skim) milk**
1/8 cup rolled oats
1 ripe banana
1/2 tsp cinnamon
1/4 tsp nutmeg
3 or 4 ice cubes

Directions

1. Slice carrot and banana.
2. Place all ingredients in a blender and blend until smooth.

Nutritional Information (per serving): Calories 127, Sodium 108mg

*Other kinds of milk such as soy, flax, or coconut may be substituted for low-fat milk.

Sweet Pea Smoothie

Peas have never tasted so sweet! This healthy recipe of peas, pineapple, banana, and strawberry makes a unique and tasty smoothie! It is perfect for a mid-morning snack, and it deliciously sneaks an additional portion of vegetables into your diet. A mid-morning snack can help you eat more frequent, smaller meals during the day to help you manage your portion size, a key for people with GERD. Just combine the ingredients in the blender, blend until smooth, and voila! We're pretty sure you won't be hungry for a big lunch!

Recipe serves 2

Ingredients

1 1/2 cup pineapple juice
1 cup frozen strawberries
1/3 cup frozen peas
1 banana

Directions

1. Cook peas according to package directions, then rinse, drain, and cool.
2. Place the cooked peas in the blender
3. Add the remaining ingredients, cover, and blend on high speed until smooth (about 30 seconds)
4. Pour the mixture into two glasses and enjoy!

Nutritional information (per serving): Calories 190, Sodium 25mg

Fruity vegetable juice

Vegetable juice might taste strange at first, but you will quickly acquire a taste for veggie drinks by adding sweet fruits like pears, kiwi, grapes, and mangoes to the mix. All of these fruits are GERD diet friendly, and pair well with a variety of veggies, including cucumber, celery, watercress, and sweet peppers - so put on your creative hat! For this drink recipe, we use broccoli and sweeten it up with pear juice, grapes, and bean sprouts. The sprouts are mild in flavor, bursting with vitamins, and juicy enough to work well in any nourishing blend. So satisfyingly good!

Yields 2 small servings

Ingredients

3 1/2 oz fresh broccoli
1 large pear
1/2 cup bean sprouts (3 1/2 oz)
7 oz green grapes
1/2 tsp shaved ginger root
1/4 tsp cinnamon

Directions

1. Cut broccoli into small pieces.
2. Quarter the pear and remove the core and chop.
3. Push all the ingredients including the sprouts through the juicer.
4. Add ginger and cinnamon, and mix well.
5. Serve immediately in glasses filled with ice cubes.

Nutritional information (per serving): Calories 119, Sodium 10mg

Butternut squash soup

This recipe is a great tasting first course that is warm, filling, packed with vitamins and minerals, and, of course, delicious – perfect for a cold winter night! The recipe sounds a little different if you're not used to using different spices, but the flavors come together wonderfully. The yellow curry powder is not spicy, but is a great flavor enhancer, and nutmeg is a secret ingredient!

Recipe serves 8-10

Ingredients

4 cloves garlic, minced
¼ cup olive oil
1 large butternut squash
4 carrots
1 parsnip
6 cups vegetable stock (low sodium)
½ tsp Paprika
1 tsp Yellow curry powder
½ tsp nutmeg
1/8 tsp Salt
½ tsp Pepper

Directions

1. Begin sautéing garlic on low with the olive oil in a large saucepan or stockpot.
2. Peel and dice the squash into 1-2" pieces, discarding the seeds and peel.
3. Slice carrots (do not peel).
4. Slice parsnips (do not peel).
5. Add carrots and parsnips to olive oil and sauté on medium for 3 minutes
6. Add squash to the pan and slowly add ½ tsp of salt and ½ tsp pepper while stirring.
7. Add 1 tsp yellow curry powder, ½ tsp nutmeg, ½ tsp paprika and stir to spread spices evenly over the vegetables let cook 5 minutes.
8. Add 6 cups vegetable stock and bring to a boil. Simmer for 15-20 minutes until squash is very tender and breakable with a fork.
9. Using a blender, puree the soup 1 cup at a time and add into a separate container. Once all is pureed and stirred, the soup it is ready to be served!
10. Put in bowls and add a small spoonful of low fat sour cream in the middle of each soup bowl for a nice presentation. Cut up some nice French or sourdough bread to dip with.

Nutritional information (per serving): Calories 124, Sodium 430mg

Chicken tortilla soup

Nothing hits the spot like a warm hearty soup on a chilly fall evening. Reduced fat tortilla chips give a nice texture to our healthy recipe of chicken tortilla soup. Top your bowl with low fat shredded Monterey Jack or Cheddar cheese. Toss a crisp iceberg lettuce salad to round out a delicious meal!

Recipe serves 4

Ingredients

3 large bone in chicken breasts
1 package frozen corn
1 large onion (sautéed to reduce acid content)
3 ribs celery sliced
3 large carrots sliced
2 tsp ground cumin
1 tsp paprika
1 tsp chili powder
7 cups water
1 1/2 TBSP olive oil
20 reduced-fat tortilla chips (crushed)
1 cup shredded reduced fat cheese (cheddar or Monterey jack)

Directions

1. To a large sauce pot, add the olive oil and sauté the chopped onion over medium heat for about 2 minutes.
2. Add sliced carrots, sliced celery and the spices to the pot. Continue to cook for 2 minutes more.
3. Pour the water into the pot, add the chicken breasts and frozen corn. Stir the mixture and bring to a simmer. Continue to simmer, stirring occasionally for 45 minutes.
4. Carefully remove the chicken from the pot and shred. Add the shredded chicken back to the pot and stir.
5. Ladle into soup bowls and top with desired amount of cheese and chips and enjoy!

Nutritional information (per serving): Calories 328, Sodium 285mg

Creamy split pea soup

Split peas are GERD friendly and packed with healthy vitamins and nutrients. This soup is delicious and perfect for a chilly evening. It's also a great way to use a leftover ham bone. We use low-sodium chicken broth in this recipe and flavor it up with lots of heartburn friendly seasonings. Be sure not to skimp on the cooking time because the peas taste best when they reach a "creamy" consistency. Enjoy!

Makes about 6 servings

Ingredients

1 ham bone
1 pound split peas
8 cups low sodium chicken broth
1 cup chopped celery
2 to 3 diced carrots
1 TBSP dried chopped onion*
1 bay leaf
1/2 tsp thyme
1/2 tsp ginger
1/2 tsp pepper
1/2 tsp marjoram
1/4 tsp dried mustard

Directions

1. Rinse peas well and inspect and pick off all debris.
2. In a large stockpot, bring chicken broth to a boil.
3. Add ham bone and simmer for 45 minutes.
4. Remove ham bone and allow to cool.
5. Add cleaned peas, all seasonings, and remaining ingredients to the pan, and return to a boil. Reduce heat to a low simmer and cover the pan. Simmer on low for at least one hour or until the peas almost disintegrate.
6. Stir often to avoid burning, and if the soup gets too thick, add more broth.
7. When ready to serve, pick the meat off the ham bone and return to the pot, stir well, and ladle into soup bowls.

*Dried chopped onions are more GERD friendly than fresh onions, but avoid them if they trigger your symptoms

Nutritional information (per serving): Calories 266, Sodium 369mg

Homemade turkey soup

The combination of a large variety of spices simmered with a leftover turkey carcass gives the broth in this popular soup recipe a unique and fabulous flavor. The turkey carcass should have at least two cups of meat remaining on it to make a good, rich soup. We keep the soup lower in saturated fat and GERD diet friendly by preparing it ahead of time, allowing it to cool, and then skimming off the fat that rises to the top. Then we add thyme, rosemary, sage, basil, marjoram, tarragon, and pepper....need we say more? Warm and wonderful!

Recipe makes about 16 1-cup servings

Ingredients

6 pound turkey breast carcass. It should have some meat (at least 2 cups) remaining on it to make a good, rich soup.
2 TBSP dried minced onions*
3 stalks of celery
1 tsp dried thyme
1/2 tsp dried rosemary
1/2 tsp dried sage
1 tsp dried basil
1/2 tsp dried marjoram
1/2 tsp dried tarragon
1/2 tsp salt
to taste black pepper
1/2 pound pasta

Directions

1. Place turkey breast in a large 6-quart pot. Cover with water, at least 3/4 full.
2. Wash celery stalks, slice, and add to pot with dried minced onion
3. Simmer covered for about 2-1/2 hours.
4. Remove carcass from pot. Divide soup into smaller, shallower containers for quick cooling in the refrigerator.
5. After cooling, skim off fat.
6. While soup is cooling, remove remaining meat from turkey carcass. Cut into pieces.
7. Add turkey meat to skimmed soup along with herbs and spices.
8. Bring to a boil and add pasta.
9. Continue cooking on low boil for about 20 minutes until pasta is done.
10. Serve at once or refrigerate for later reheating.

Nutritional information (per serving): Calories 226, Sodium 217mg

Fresh Vegetable and White Bean Soup

There is nothing more satisfying than a warm and hearty bowl of soup on a winter night. This recipe is a healthy, low-sodium, low-fat version of a favorite soup, made with "no sodium" chicken broth and just a bit of regular vegetable bouillon. What makes the broth delicious is the combination of fresh vegetables simmered together with the white beans. You can also add some shredded cooked chicken (or ham) to the finished soup for a complete meal. Then stoke up the fire and enjoy!

Makes four 3/4 cup servings

Ingredients

3 TBSP chopped white onion
1 cup sliced fresh mushrooms
1/2 cup julienned carrots (or sliced)
1 cup fresh broccoli florets
1 cup fresh cauliflower florets
2 large celery stalks sliced
1 can Northern beans (14 ounce), drained and rinsed
2 TBSP no sodium chicken broth
1/2 TBSP "Better than Bouillon" vegetable broth
1 TBSP olive oil
2 1/2 cups water
2 TBSP red or white wine
1/4 tsp garlic salt
Parmesan cheese (optional)

Directions

1. Spray nonstick pan with cooking spray.
2. Add olive oil and heat to medium.
3. Add vegetables and sauté on low heat for 4 minutes. Do not overcook.
4. Add water, bouillon, garlic salt, and white beans.
5. Simmer on low until veggies are cooked "al dente," about another 10 minutes.
6. Ladle into bowls and top with a little Parmesan cheese. Enjoy!

Nutritional information (per serving): Calories 99, Sodium 175mg

Vegetable chowder

The term "chowder" comes from the word "chaudiere" which is the French word for cauldron, the pot in which thick stews and soups are cooked in France. Most Americans will first think of clam chowder, but chowders are actually a broad range of soups that typically use flour for thickening. To keep our recipe GERD diet friendly, we didn't include flour and thickened it up instead with chunky potatoes, broccoli, cream of celery soup, and cream style yellow corn. Season this mixture with some ginger and parsley, and you will have a yummy and comforting cold weather soup.

Yields 4 (1 cup) servings

Ingredients

1 can reduced fat cream of celery soup (10-3/4 oz)
1 cup fat free milk
1-1/2 cups cooked potatoes (diced)
1 cup cream style yellow corn, without salt added
1 cup broccoli (thawed from frozen)
1 teaspoon dried onion flakes*
1/2 tsp ginger
1 tsp parsley

Directions

1. Combine soup, milk, cream corn, dried onion, and seasonings in a large saucepan.
2. Mix well and stir in broccoli and potatoes.
3. Bring the mixture to a boil, while stirring often.
4. Reduce the heat and bring to a slow simmer.
5. Cover the pan and cook for about 15 more minutes, stirring occasionally.

Nutritional information: 240 calories, Sodium 720mg

*Omit onion if the dried form triggers your GERD symptoms.

Cauliflower soup

Cauliflower has some fantastic health benefits: it is low in calories, high in fiber and vitamin C, and contains a broad spectrum of antioxidant nutrients. Cauliflower is also considered a safe vegetable for people following a GERD diet. When selecting a cauliflower, look for a clean, creamy white head, surrounded by many thick green leaves. They are better protected and will be fresher. Spotted or dull colored cauliflower should be avoided. This puréed soup is healthy and delicious and perfect for cool nights! Warm and wonderful!

Recipe makes 4 1-cup servings

Ingredients

1 medium head of cauliflower, cut up
4 cups low sodium chicken broth
1/3 cup uncooked brown rice
1/2 cup finely chopped celery
1/2 tsp ginger
1 T soft margarine
1/2 cup low fat milk
1/8 t kosher salt
1/4 t pepper
1 T dried onion*

Directions

1. Cook cauliflower, rice, and celery in boiling broth until rice is tender.
2. Add spices.
3. Remove from stove and add milk.
4. Purée in blender.
5. Serve hot or cold.

*Dried onion is optional, and can be included if it does not trigger your heartburn symptoms.

Nutritional information (per serving): Calories 104, Sodium 25mg

Chicken noodle soup

Nothing is more comforting in cold weather than a warm bowl of chicken soup! And besides comfort, folklore has given chicken soup a reputation as a remedy for colds and flu. This easy recipe makes a hearty meal using precooked chicken meat, whole wheat pasta noodles, and three different vegetables. For the GERD diet friendly base, we mix together reduced fat cream of chicken soup, nonfat dry milk, and low sodium chicken broth seasoned with parsley and ginger. It's filling and delicious, and it just might "cure what ails you!"

Recipe makes 4 servings

Ingredients

1 cup chopped celery
1 cup shredded carrots
1 can reduced fat cream of chicken soup
1/3 cup nonfat dry milk powder
1 (14 ounce) can low sodium chicken broth
1 tsp dried parsley flakes
1/2 tsp ginger
1 TBSP dried minced onion (optional)
1 1/2 cups cooked chicken (diced)
1/2 cup frozen peas
1 cup uncooked wide egg noodles (whole wheat)

Directions

1. Spray a saucepan with butter flavored nonstick cooking spray and sauté the carrots and celery for six minutes.
2. Stir in next five ingredients, including the optional dried onion*, and mix well.
3. Add chicken and peas.
4. Mix well and continue cooking the soup for about 7 minutes, stirring occasionally.
5. In a separate pot, cook the egg noodles in water according to directions.
6. Serve the soup hot and add desired amount of noodles.

*Omit dried onion if they trigger your GERD symptoms.

Nutritional information (per serving): Calories 237, Sodium 560mg

Picnic potato salad

Nothing is more essential for a summer picnic than a delicious potato salad. This "All-American" fresh vegetable dish is mayo-based and seasoned with savory spices to give it a lot of zest. Yukon gold, fingerling, or red bliss potatoes will work best for this recipe because they keep their shape well when cooked. Be sure not to overcook the potatoes and to remove them from heat while still slightly firm. We also recommend seasoning the potatoes while still warm so that they better absorb the flavors. It's low in fat, GERD diet friendly, and simply mouthwatering!

Makes 10 1/2-cup servings

Ingredients

6 medium peeled* potatoes (about 2 lbs)
3 stalks celery, finely chopped
1/3 cup red bell pepper, coarsely chopped
1 TBSP dried minced onion**
1 egg hard boiled, chopped
6 TBSP light mayonnaise
1 tsp Dijon mustard
1/2 tsp salt
1/4 tsp black pepper
1/4 tsp dill weed, dried
1/4 tsp ginger, dried

Directions

1. Wash and peel potatoes, cut in half, and place them in cold water in a saucepan.
2. Cook covered over medium heat for 25 to 30 minutes or until tender.
3. Remove from heat and drain well. Season with salt, pepper, ginger, and dill.
4. Evenly dice potatoes when cool.
5. Add vegetables and egg to potatoes and toss.
6. Blend together mayonnaise and Dijon mustard.
7. Pour dressing over potato mixture and stir gently to coat evenly.
8. Chill for at least 1 hour before serving.

Nutritional information (per serving): Calories 98, Sodium 212mg

*If you prefer unpeeled potatoes, be sure to scrub and clean the skins well, and be aware that they do not absorb the flavors as well as peeled potatoes.

**Omit the dried minced onion if they trigger your GERD symptoms

Sunshine pasta salad

This cold pasta salad recipe serves a crowd, so it's perfect for a big family picnic or a summer cookout. We prepare the dish a day ahead and place it in the fridge to marinate overnight. This gives it a unique and tasty "sweet and sour" flavor. We then drain the marinade from the pasta and vegetables prior to serving, which keeps them lower in fat and GERD diet friendly. When ready to serve, just place a few tablespoons of the mixture on each lettuce leaf. You will relish the sunny flavors!

Makes 18 1/2 cup servings

Ingredients

16 oz uncooked small seashell macaroni (9 cups cooked)
2 TBSP vegetable oil
3/4 cup sugar
1/2 cup apple cider vinegar
1/2 cup wine vinegar
1/2 cup water
3 TBSP prepared mustard
1/4 tsp black pepper
2 oz jar pimentos
2 small cucumbers
2 stalks celery
18 Lettuce leaves

Directions

1. Cook shells in unsalted water, drain, rinse with cold water, and drain again.
2. Transfer shells to 4-quart bowl, and stir in oil.
3. Place sugar, vinegars, water, prepared mustard, salt, pepper, and pimento into a blender.
4. Process at low speed for 15-20 seconds, or just enough so flecks of pimento can be seen.
5. Pour over macaroni.
6. Cut cucumber in half lengthwise, then thinly slice.
7. Chop and dice celery.
8. Add to pasta and toss well.
9. Marinate, covered, in refrigerator for 24 hours. Stir occasionally.
10. Drain the mixture well and serve on lettuce slices.

Nutritional information (per serving): Calories 149, Sodium 33mg

Asian noodle salad

Rice vermicelli is a delicate form of rice noodle that is commonly used in recipes throughout China and Southeast Asia. They are thin and tender and although they don't have much taste on their own, they readily absorb the flavors of the foods and spices they are cooked with. Commonly used in soups and stir-fry, the noodles also make a nice addition to a salad, so give this recipe a try. The noodles are fat free, cholesterol free, and low in sodium, which makes them a healthy addition to your GERD friendly diet! They are easy to prepare and for convenience can be made up to two days ahead and stored in the refrigerator. Enjoy!

Yields 4 servings

Ingredients

6 ounces vermicelli rice noodles
1/4 cup rice vinegar
2 tsp sugar
1 1/2 TBSP fresh grated ginger
1 red bell pepper seeded and sliced
3 oz. snow peas trimmed and sliced lengthwise
1/2 English cucumber sliced and cut into half moons
1 TBSP Vegetable or canola oil
1 lb. lean ground pork, chicken or turkey
1/4 cup hoisin sauce
1 finely chopped large celery stalk

Directions

1. Cook the vermicelli according to package directions. Rinse with cold water to cool, drain well, and set aside.
2. In a large bowl, mix together vinegar, 1 tsp ginger, and 1/4 tsp salt. Stir in the snow peas, peppers, cucumbers, and celery.
3. Add the oil to a large nonstick skillet and heat to medium. Add the ground meat and cook thoroughly. Stir in the hoisin sauce and remaining ginger. Add 2 TBSP water and cook for 1 additional minute.
4. Evenly divide the cooled noodles onto 4 plates and top with the ground meat mixture and the prepared salad.

Nutritional information (per serving): Calories 454, Sodium 445mg

Dijon chicken salad

We like to make the chicken from scratch for this recipe using bone-in chicken breasts poached gently in salted water, but you can also use leftovers or pre-cooked white chicken meat for this salad. The white peaches add just the right sweetness, and shredded carrots and red cabbage make this a healthy and tasty lunch or light dinner. The low-calorie Dijon herb vinaigrette is seasoned with your choice of acid reflux diet friendly spices, so choose your favorite, and enjoy!

Yields 4 servings

Ingredients

2 large chicken breasts on the bone
2 large white peaches, peeled and chopped
1/2 cup shredded carrots
1 cup shredded red cabbage (or finely chopped broccoli)

4 large Romaine or Bibb lettuce leaves
2 TBSP Gorgonzola cheese crumbles (feta or goat)
3 TBSP toasted chopped walnuts

Directions

1. Place the chicken breasts in a large stockpot and cover with water. Salt the water and heat to a simmer. Poach the chicken gently until done about 30 minutes. Do not boil the water. Remove from water and let cool.
2. Shred the cooled chicken and add it to a mixing bowl with the peaches, carrots, and cabbage.
3. Make the salad dressing and set aside. *
4. Place the 4 lettuce leaves on salad plates and divide the chicken salad evenly on the leaves.
5. Spoon desired amount of vinaigrette on the salad.
6. Top with cheese and chopped walnuts.

*Dijon Herb Vinaigrette

Whisk together 3 T of Champagne or red wine vinegar, 1 T of Dijon mustard, 1 T of finely chopped parsley, and 1 T of finely chopped fresh basil, ginger, marjoram, or thyme. Slowly add in 1/3 cup of extra virgin olive oil and season with a dash of salt and pepper.

If you use a prepared vinaigrette, be sure to read the label carefully to avoid dressings that are high in sugar or trans fats. Choose those that are made with extra virgin olive oil or canola oil, and be aware that low-fat and non-fat dressings have added sugar to make them more flavorful.

Nutritional information (per serving - approximate): Calories 311, Sodium 310mg

Healthy hodgepodge salad

No time to cook? Take a look in your pantry and fridge to see what you have on hand that's healthy and also GERD friendly. We found canned tuna, white beans, walnuts, and brown rice in the pantry, and in the fridge we had feta cheese, fresh beets, lettuce, carrots, and a hard boiled egg. While this isn't a traditional recipe, a "hodgepodge" meal like this is fun, so be creative! It works with a myriad of ingredients including cabbage, kale, arugula, mushrooms, quinoa, celery, avocado - whatever you have readily available. You can also add leftover chicken, steak or fish. Just put all the ingredients together in a large bowl, toss with your favorite low fat salad dressing, and voila! It's ready to go in just minutes!

Makes about 2 servings

Ingredients

1 can solid white albacore tuna (7 oz)
1/2 cup white kidney or garbanzo beans
2 fresh beets (packaged)
1 large carrot
1 cup cooked brown rice
2 cups mixed greens
1 hard boiled egg*
1/4 cup walnuts
Low fat sesame salad dressing
Feta cheese

Directions

1. Drain and flake the tuna.
2. Drain beans well.
3. Slice the carrot, beets, and hard boiled egg.
4. Place the mixed greens in a large bowl and top with tuna, beans, carrots, beets, walnuts, and feta cheese.
5. Toss with desired amount of salad dressing.
6. Put the lettuce mixture into individual bowls, and top with egg slices.

For nutritional information when making your own "healthy hodgepodge" use the "food search" at www.calorieking.com and type in your choice of ingredients.

*Omit the egg if it triggers your GERD symptoms.

Baby Kale and Edamame Salad

We all know that vegetables are very, very good for our bodies, but even with that knowledge, most of us do not include enough greens in our diet. This GERD-friendly salad is a nutritious and delicious addition to your acid reflux diet plan. For those not familiar with kale, it is known as the "queen of greens," and it has recently become a shining star in the salad category. Kale, like broccoli and brussel sprouts, is a member of the cabbage family and it contains an abundance of nutrients, including beta carotene, calcium, vitamins C and B6, folic acid, manganese, and potassium. We use organic baby kale in our heartburn-friendly salad to make the preparation quick and easy. A healthy trio of cucumber, edamame, and red cabbage completes the recipe and is tossed with a generous amount of our own GERD-friendly apricot ginger vinaigrette and topped with raisins and slivered almonds. Give it a try! We think you will savor the flavor!

Serves 4 to 6

Ingredients

For the salad:

1 pkg. organic baby kale (10 oz)*

1/2 cup edamame beans

1 cup shredded red cabbage

1 whole cucumber thinly sliced

1/4 cup slivered almonds

1/4 cup raisins

3 TBSP feta cheese (optional)

For the apricot vinaigrette:

1/4 cup olive oil

1/4 cup apricot preserves

1 1/2 TBSP apple cider vinegar

1 TBSP water

1/2 tsp ginger

1 pinch of both pepper and sea salt

Directions

1. Place the kale in a salad bowl.
2. Prepare vinaigrette. Combine all ingredients listed for the vinaigrette in a mixing bowl and whisk well.
3. Mix 6 TBSP of vinaigrette into the kale. Toss until well coated.
4. Set the coated kale aside for 10 minutes, so it starts to wilt.
5. Add the sliced cucumbers, edamame, shredded cabbage, almonds, and raisins to the bowl and toss the mixture well with the remaining vinaigrette.
6. If desired top with a sprinkle of feta.

*You can substitute the baby kale for 2 bunches of curly kale. The leaves need to be trimmed of stems, washed and dried and then shredded into bite size pieces.

Nutritional information (per serving): Calories 310, Sodium 110mg

Shrimpy Spinach Salad

All the experts these days seem to agree that eating fish is good for your health. This salad recipe is GERD friendly and one of our favorites, and it's a creative way to add a little extra seafood to your diet. The combination of shrimp, strawberries, and asparagus is perfectly paired with raspberry vinaigrette and topped for crunch with slivered almonds. The dish is low in calories, but filling, so it makes a great lunch or light dinner. Better yet, we think it might even satisfy your sweet tooth too!

Makes four servings

Ingredients

12 large cooked shrimp
1/2 cup low fat raspberry vinaigrette (divided)
5 cups chopped baby spinach leaves
1/3 cup slivered almonds (unsalted)
8 ripe fresh strawberries (sliced)
8 cooked and cooled asparagus spears (trimmed of rough ends) and cut in half
4 Tablespoons Bleu cheese* (optional)

Directions

1. Marinate the cooked shrimp in 1/4 cup vinaigrette for 20 minutes in the refrigerator.
2. Remove shrimp after 20 minutes and discard vinaigrette.
3. Place the spinach leaves in a large bowl and toss with remaining 1/4 cup raspberry vinaigrette
4. Divide the leaves equally onto four plates.
5. Top the leaves with the shrimp, strawberries, and asparagus.
6. Sprinkle with slivered almonds and top with 1 Tablespoon Bleu cheese.

Nutritional Information: Calories 254, Sodium 116mg

*1 TBSP Bleu cheese = 18 Calories and 95mg Sodium

Whole Wheat Pasta Salad

Most of us think of pasta salad and we think of lots of mayonnaise. While that may taste great, the after effects from all that heavy saturated fat may not be worth it when you suffer from reflux disease! So, here is a recipe for a light summer pasta salad that is healthy and tastes great. It replaces the mayo with vinaigrette and uses herbs and feta cheese to enhance the flavor. This recipe calls for cherry tomatoes. They are less acidic and slightly sweeter than regular tomatoes and are often tolerated by people with reflux disease; however, it they bother you, try replacing them with red grapes.

Recipe serves 10 (1 cup per serving)

Ingredients

16 oz, 1 box of whole wheat rotini pasta
3 TBSP red or white wine vinegar (balsamic works too if you want it sweeter)
1 TBSP lemon juice (if you can tolerate lemon, otherwise an extra T of vinegar will work)
½ cup extra virgin olive oil
1 ¼ lb cherry tomatoes, halved
1 cup green onion or chives chopped
½ cup pitted kalamata olives sliced
½ cup chopped basil
½ cup chopped parsley
1 cup crumbled goat or feta cheese
Salt & pepper to taste

Directions

1. Cook pasta al dente, according to package directions.
2. Once finished, rinse pasta and let drain well before transferring to a large bowl.
3. While pasta is cooking, mix vinegar and lemon. Slowly add oil while stirring continuously to ensure thorough mixture.
4. Pour the dressing over the pasta.
5. Mix in the herbs, tomato, and cheese.
6. Add salt and pepper to taste.
7. Best if served at room temperature of chilled.

Nutritional information (per serving): Calories 405, Sodium 232mg

Cucumber Salad

Cucumbers have some terrific health benefits, so making them a part of your regular GERD-friendly diet is a smart choice. It's easy too! You can eat sliced cucumbers for an afternoon snack, use them as a sandwich topping, and include them in any of your salads. This refreshing recipe is easy to prepare and will last up to a week in the refrigerator. We like to make this a day ahead, because the longer it marinates, the tastier it is. It's a perfect blend of tart and sweetness, so be healthy and give it a try!

Makes 8 servings

Ingredients

2 cups white vinegar
1 cup water
1/2 cup sugar (or adjusted amount of sugar substitute)
1 tsp Kosher Salt*
1/4 cup fresh or dried dill weed
4 large firm cucumbers, thinly sliced
1 stalk celery, thinly sliced
1 carrot, scraped and thinly sliced

Directions

1. The day before serving, bring vinegar, water, sugar, and dill to a boil.
2. Meanwhile, layer the vegetables in a medium sized bowl.
3. Pour the boiling vinegar mixture over the vegetables.
4. Cover, cool, and then refrigerate overnight.
5. Serve cold in small fruit dishes.

Nutritional information (per serving): Calories 55, Sodium 245mg

*To keep this recipe to 2.6mg of sodium, omit the Kosher salt.

GERD-friendly Salad Dressings

Salads are excellent on *RefluxMD's Recipe for Relief*, but unfortunately, many prepared salad dressing are terrible for you. Most have too many calories, too much sodium, and too many saturated fats. We put this list together to allow everyone to not only eat a healthy salad, but enjoy it as well.

Vinaigrette Salad Dressing

Mix 1/2 cup water with 1/4 tsp ginger, 1 TBSP Red Wine Vinegar, and 1/4 tsp honey. Whisk in 1 TBSP virgin olive oil and 1/4 tsp black pepper. Yields 4 (2 TBSP) servings.

Calories 33, Sodium 0mg

Creamy Yogurt Salad Dressing

Mix 8 oz fat free plain yogurt with 1/4 cup fat free mayonnaise. Add 2 TBSP dried dill weed, 1 TBSP ginger, cilantro or basil, and 2 TBSP apple cider vinegar. Whisk well and refrigerate. Yields 8 (2 TBSP) servings.

Calories 23, Sodium 84mg

Apricot Vinaigrette

Mix 1/4 Cup olive oil with 1/4 Cup sugar free apricot preserves. Add 1 1/2 TBSP Apple Cider or Rice Wine Vinegar, 1 TBSP water and 1/2 tsp ginger. Whisk until well mixed. Yields 5 (2 TBSP) servings.

Calories 110, Sodium 0mg

Dijon Herb Vinaigrette

Mix 3 TBSP champagne or white wine vinegar with 1 TBSP Dijon mustard. Add 1 TBSP finely chopped parsley, 1 TBSP fresh basil or ginger and 1 TBSP marjoram or thyme. Slowly whisk in 1/3 cup Extra Virgin Olive oil. Yields 6 (2 TBSP) Servings.

Calories 102, Sodium 56mg

Marinated Mushroom Sandwich

In this recipe, mushrooms are the stars instead of meat because the end result is lower in fat, making this sandwich easier to digest. Olive oil is used instead of butter or other fats like mayonnaise because it contains essential healthy fats with almost no saturated fat. The feta cheese is strong in flavor, so it provides the satisfaction of cheese, but not much is needed. Mixing the cheese with basil and olive oil makes a faux pesto aioli with less calories and fat then if mayonnaise had been used, further lowering the overall fat content.

Recipe serves 4

Ingredients

1 package pre cut mushrooms usually 8 oz (Either Portobello or crimini mushrooms will work for this recipe.)
2 TBSP olive oil
1 TBSP Worcestershire sauce
3 cloves garlic- finely chopped
1 dash salt and/or pepper to taste
1 tsp thyme
4 ciabatta rolls
½ cup crumbled feta cheese
10 fresh basil leaves
1 tsp olive oil
4 cups baby spinach

Directions

1. Place mushrooms, olive oil, Worcestershire sauce, garlic, salt and thyme in a gallon bag and let marinade for a minimum of an hour. Every so often shake the mushrooms around inside the closed bag to allow maximum absorption.
2. While the mushrooms marinate, chop the basil leaves and place them in a bowl. Add 1 tsp olive oil and ½ cup feta to the chopped basil and stir.
3. After marinating, place mushrooms on a cookie sheet and broil on high for 3 minutes. Flip the mushrooms and broil for 3 more minutes.
4. While broiling the mushrooms, toast the ciabatta rolls.
5. Spread feta and basil mixture thinly across one half of a roll and put mushrooms and spinach on top. If you can tolerate tomato you can also add sliced tomato. Or if you are feeling adventurous, marinated artichoke hearts are great with this sandwich, too.

Nutritional information (per serving): Calories 295, Sodium 200mg

Lentil Burgers

Why lentils? Lentils are delicious and versatile enough to make a tasty and healthy version of a "hamburger," they are filling, but low in calories and contain virtually no fat, and last but not least, lentils are GERD friendly and do not promote heartburn! Serve alone or on a whole wheat bun with iceberg lettuce and honey mustard. Mmm Mmm delightful!

Serves 4

Ingredients

2 cups cooked lentils
1/2 cup dried breadcrumbs
1/2 cup egg beaters
1/4 cup grated carrot
3/4 cup chopped kale*
1 or 2 TBSP chopped dried onion (according to preference)
1/4 tsp kosher salt
1/2 tsp pepper
1/2 tsp cumin
1/3 cup grated sharp cheddar cheese
Iceberg lettuce
Honey mustard dressing
Whole wheat hamburger buns (toasted)
1 TBSP Canola or olive oil

Directions

1. Combine together the cooked lentils, breadcrumbs, egg beaters (or two egg whites), and cheese with the chopped kale, carrots, and dried onion. Add the spices and form into four 3/4-inch patties. Do not add the oil. Chill burgers well for at least 1 hour on a wax paper lined baking sheet.
2. When ready to cook, pour the oil into a nonstick skillet and heat until bubbly. Add the chilled burgers and reduce heat to medium. Set a timer for 2 1/2 minutes. Flip over when the timer goes off and continue to cook for an additional 2 to 3 minutes or until the burgers look browned and are piping hot!
3. Lightly drain the patties on paper towels, and then serve on toasted buns with iceberg lettuce and honey mustard dressing.

*Fresh chopped spinach can be substituted for chopped kale

Nutritional information (per burger): Calories 252, Sodium 394mg

Vegan chia burger

Chia is a tiny little seed with big nutrition including iron, omega 3, magnesium, calcium, and selenium. WOW! On top of that, chia is known to give a full feeling, which can help you avoid overeating - a key factor for a successful GERD diet. The seeds are easy to add to a wide variety of recipes including soups, sauces, smoothies, and burgers. We combined chia seeds with sunflower seeds, chopped almonds, and coconut oil to give this vegan burger a pleasant "nutty" flavor. It's tasty, sweet, and so unique!

Yields 6 servings and can easily be doubled to make 12

Ingredients

2 1/2 TBSP chia seeds

1/2 cup water

1 tsp coconut oil

1 tsp cumin

1 tsp ginger

1/2 tsp oregano

1/8 cup chopped cilantro

1/4 cup finely chopped and diced celery

9 oz reduced sodium black beans (canned, rinsed and drained)

1 TBSP sesame oil

1/4 cup chopped almonds

1/2 cup chopped sunflower seeds (dry roasted without salt)

1 1/2 cups plain breadcrumbs

1/4 cup low sodium soy sauce

1 cup grated carrots

1 cup oats

Flour for dredging

1 to 2 TBSP coconut oil for cooking

Directions

1. Mix chia seeds and water in a small bowl. Let seeds soak for 6 minutes until they have absorbed the water. The texture will be syrupy and similar to a raw egg yolk.
2. Sauté the celery in coconut oil and then remove from pan and place in a large mixing bowl to cool.
3. When the celery is cooled, add the chia, seasonings, and all the remaining ingredients to the bowl.
4. Mix well and shape into 6 patties.
5. Dredge patties in flour.
6. Heat 1 TBSP coconut oil over medium heat in a large skillet. Cook burgers in batches of 3 until they are golden brown on each side and heated through, adding remaining coconut oil as needed.

Nutritional information (per serving): Calories 295, Sodium 630mg

Salmon Burgers with Miso Yogurt and Carrot Slaw

If you like crab cakes, you will enjoy these salmon burgers because they are just as tasty and have a similar flaky texture. This is an Asian-inspired recipe that is made with fresh ginger and white miso, which are both considered GERD-friendly spices. For those not familiar with white miso, it's a traditional Japanese seasoning, in paste form, made from fermented soybeans. We mix the white miso paste with plain yogurt to make a delicious low-fat, mayonnaise-style topping for the burger. A tablespoon or two of our own carrot slaw finishes the sandwich, so we recommend a sturdy and lightly toasted hamburger style bun. It's very healthy and so de"lite"ful!

Serves 4

Ingredients

2 carrots grated
1 celery stalk finely chopped**
1 large egg
2 tsp rice vinegar
1 tsp canola oil
1 1/4 pound skinless salmon filet
1 TBSP finely grated fresh ginger
1 TBSP dried minced onion (optional)
1/2 cup Panko bread crumbs
1/4 cup plain yogurt
1 tsp white miso*
4 whole wheat hamburger buns
Sea or kosher salt and pepper

Directions

1. Mix together the carrots, celery**, vinegar and oil in a small bowl, and set aside.
2. Carefully cut the skinless salmon fillet into 1-inch pieces.
3. In a separate bowl, gently "hand mix" the salmon chunks, fresh ginger, bread crumbs, large egg, 1/4 tsp salt and 1/4 tsp pepper, and optional dried minced onion until the mixture is combined.
4. Form the mixture into four 3/4 inch patties and then make a small indentation with your thumb into the top of each patty. This will help prevent over-plumping during cooking.
5. Cover the patties and chill in the refrigerator for 30 minutes to 1 hour.
6. Lightly oil a clean grill and cook the patties on medium high for 8 to 10 minutes, gently flipping once at the halfway point until patties look opaque. Toast the buns on the grill.

7. Place the cooked patties onto the prepared buns, and top each with a tablespoon or more of miso yogurt (recipe follows) and the desired amount of carrot slaw.

Miso Yogurt

Mix 1/4 cup plain yogurt with 1 teaspoon white miso* (soybean paste) until combined.

*White miso can be found in the refrigerated section of your grocery store

**If sweet peppers are not one of your trigger foods, you can substitute 1/4 cup finely chopped red or green peppers for the celery, if desired.

Nutritional information (per serving): Calories 410, Sodium 619mg

Hawaiian-style Ahi Sandwich with Coconut Slaw

Want a taste of the tropics on a cold winter day? Let your taste buds transport you to Hawaii with our acid reflux-friendly fish sandwich. Ahi tuna, also called yellowfin, is one of the largest of the tuna species. In fact, one of the record catches of yellowfin tuna was measured at a whopping 300 pounds! Wow! Yet despite its girth, yellowfin tuna is surprisingly low in fat. It is also is a great source of several nutrients you need for good health including protein, potassium, phosphorous, and vitamins D and B-12. These recipes are easy and fun to prepare and we think you will savor the island flavors. Be sure to use a sturdy whole wheat hamburger style bun for the sandwich and spread it generously with our own RefluxMD "tropical" pineapple mustard. Aloha!

Ahi Sandwich

Serves 2

Ingredients

Two 3 to 4 oz* portions ahi tuna steaks (washed and dried)
1/2 tsp dried thyme mixed with 1/2 tsp olive oil
Two large romaine lettuce leaves
Two whole wheat hamburger style buns
1 TBSP canned crushed pineapple (well drained)
1 TBSP Dijon mustard
1 tsp Honey
1/8 tsp White pepper

Directions

1. Preheat oven to 350 degrees.
2. Prepare the "tropical" mustard by combining the pineapple, dijon mustard, honey, and white pepper. Mix well and set aside.
3. Rub the tuna with the oil and thyme mixture.
4. Place tuna in the oven (preferably on a glass dish) and cook for approximately 20 minutes. Check for desired (rare to medium) doneness.
5. Spread on each bun the tropical mustard.
6. Place the fish and lettuce on the prepared buns and serve immediately.

Nutritional information: Calories 362, Sodium 173mg

*Let your own appetite be the judge for portion size because the nutritional value variance for this dish is insignificant.

Coconut Coleslaw
Makes 4 one cup servings

Ingredients
2 cups cabbage
1 cup shredded carrot
1/2 apple (chopped)
1/3 cup crushed canned pineapple (well drained)
3/4 cup coconut flakes
1/4 cup raisins
1/2 tsp Dijon mustard
1/2 tsp balsamic vinegar
1/2 tsp apple cider vinegar
1/2 cup nonfat plain yogurt
1 TBSP mayonnaise
2 TBSP finely chopped parsley or cilantro
Walnuts

Directions
1. Mix carrots, cabbage, and apples together in a large bowl.
2. Add the yogurt, vinegars, mayo, and mustard, and mix well.
3. Add pineapple and coconut flakes and stir.
4. Transfer to plates, and sprinkle the portions with cilantro or parsley.
5. Top with finely chopped walnuts.

Grilled mushroom quesadilla

You don't have to go to a Mexican Restaurant to enjoy a delicious quesadilla. This GERD diet friendly recipe is a snap to make at home. A quesadilla is like a "south of the border" grilled cheese sandwich. You can fill the tortilla with a variety of low fat cheese types and add ingredients such as shredded chicken, avocado, red bell pepper, black beans, corn, and shrimp. It's easy to assemble, and the melted cheese will hold the filling in place. We fire up the grill for this low-fat recipe, but you can also use a large frying pan. Just add a scant amount of oil to the pan, and cook the tortillas over medium heat until the cheese melts, about 3 minutes per side. It's a quick lunch or dinner entree or a perfect appetizer for company. Muy muy Bueno!

Yields 4 servings

Ingredients

1 avocado, cut into half inch pieces

1 cucumber, sliced and quartered

2 TBSP olive oil

2 TBSP rice wine vinegar*

1/2 cup fresh cilantro

4 medium whole wheat flour tortillas

4 to 6 ounces** Swiss cheese

4 cups baby spinach

4 medium portobello mushroom caps

Low fat sour cream

Pepper to taste

Directions

1. Heat grill to medium.
2. Mix together the avocado, cucumber, and vinegar with 1 TBSP oil.
3. Fold in Cilantro.
4. Place the 4 tortillas on a large rimmed baking sheet. Divide half the cheese evenly among the tortillas, sprinkling it only on one half. Top that same half with spinach and remaining cheese.
5. Place the mushrooms on a cutting board and brush with remaining oil, season with pepper, and grill until tender about 3 to 4 minutes per side.
6. Divide and evenly top the mushrooms on the cheese and fold the tortillas over to cover the filling. Grill the folded tortillas for 2 minutes and flip and grill for two more minutes. Cut into wedges and serve with the avocado and cucumber mixture and if desired, a dash of sour cream.

*You can substitute lemon or lime juice for the same amount of rice wine vinegar if they do not trigger your GERD symptoms. ** If you opt for another type of cheese, go to http://www.calorieking.com/ to calculate nutritional information.

Nutritional information (per serving): Calories 422, Sodium 670mg

Pasta Primavera with Whole Wheat Pasta

Alfredo sauce for people with GERD? It sounds crazy, but this adaptation of traditional family recipe provides all of the flavor without all of the fat, so you can enjoy this dish without paying for it later. Even though this is a lighter version of a traditional dish, it has plenty of protein and fiber to keep you full. It also has many B vitamins and iron from the whole grains, calcium from the milk and butter substitute, Vitamin D in the mushrooms and dairy, and the asparagus is high in both vitamins K and A.

Recipe serves 8

Ingredients

16 oz, 1 box of whole wheat linguini pasta
4 cloves garlic
8 oz sliced porcini mushrooms
1 bunch asparagus chopped
16 oz condensed nonfat or low-fat milk unsweetened (not reconstituted)
2 TBSP butter substitute
¼ tsp nutmeg
¼ tsp salt
¼ cup Parmesan cheese
¼ cup pine nuts

Directions

1. Cook pasta al dente, as package directions instruct. Once finished let drain in a colander.
2. While the pasta is cooking chop the garlic, mushrooms, and asparagus. Heat 1 t. olive oil in a pan over medium heat. Add vegetables and sauté until tender.
3. To make the sauce, add condensed milk, butter substitute, nutmeg, and salt to a saucepan and cook on low for 5-10 minutes until it begins to thicken, stirring occasionally.
4. Once the sauce has thickened, turn off heat, add pasta, and stir until the pasta is coated.
5. To serve, place pasta on a plate, top with vegetables, and sprinkle pine nuts and Parmesan cheese on top.

Nutritional information (per serving): Calories 316, Sodium 190mg

"Guilt-free" chicken and dumplings

White skinless chicken meat and cornmeal dumplings are the basis for this low fat, yet still scrumptious GERD diet friendly stew. The recipe is made with low fat milk, onions, celery, carrots and sweet peas, and seasoned with a variety of heartburn friendly herbs. The tender dumplings are our favorite part of the dish - and the key is to not peek into the pan while they are cooking! The dumplings need to gently steam in the simmering stew to result in just the right "light" texture. It's a soulful satisfying classic!

Recipe makes 6 servings

Ingredients

For the stew:

1 pound skinless, boneless chicken meat, cut into 1-inch cubes
1/2 cup onion, coarsely chopped*
1 medium carrot, peeled and thinly sliced
1 stalk celery, thinly sliced
1/4 tsp salt
Black pepper to taste
1 pinch ground cloves
1 bay leaf
3 cups of water
1 tsp cornstarch
1 tsp dried basil
1 package (10 oz) frozen peas

For the cornmeal dumplings:

1 cup of yellow cornmeal
3/4 cup of sifted all-purpose flour
2 tsp baking powder
1/2 tsp salt
1 cup of low-fat (1%) milk
1 TBSP vegetable oil

Directions

Directions for the stew:

1. Place chicken, onion*, carrot, celery, salt, pepper, cloves, bay leaf, and water in a large saucepan.
2. Heat to boiling; cover and reduce heat to simmer. Cook about 1/2 hour or until chicken is tender.
3. Remove chicken and vegetables from broth. Strain broth.
4. Skim fat from broth; measure and, if necessary, add water to make 3 cups liquid.
5. Mix cornstarch with 1 cup cooled broth by shaking vigorously in a jar with a tight-fitting lid.
6. Pour into saucepan with remaining broth; cook, stirring constantly, until mixture comes to a boil and is thickened.
7. Add basil, peas, and reserved vegetables to sauce; stir to combine.
8. Add chicken and heat slowly to boiling while preparing cornmeal dumplings.

Directions for the dumplings:

1. Sift together cornmeal, flour, baking powder, and salt into a large mixing bowl.
2. Mix together milk and oil.
3. Add milk mixture all at once to dry ingredients; stir just enough to moisten flour and evenly distribute liquid. Dough will be soft.
4. Drop by full tablespoons on top of braised meat or stew.
5. Cover tightly; heat to boiling. Reduce heat (do not lift cover) to simmering and steam about 20 minutes.

*Omit onion if cooked onion triggers your GERD symptoms, or replace it with an appropriate amount of the dried form.

Nutritional information (per serving): Calories 307, Sodium 471mg

California fried chicken

Some California dreamers are all about staying healthy and looking good at the beach, but even the biggest "health nuts" occasionally want to indulge in some delicious fried chicken. This lightened up chicken recipe is baked in the oven, rather than fried, to keep it GERD diet friendly. We keep it even lower in fat by using vegetable oil, skim milk, and cornflakes for the breading. The flavor is ramped up with lots of seasonings, including ginger, a heartburn friendly spice. Your family will love this finger lickin' California chicken!

Recipe makes 6 servings

Ingredients

½ cup skim milk
1 tsp poultry seasoning
1 cup cornflakes, crumbled
1½ TBSP onion powder
1 ½ TBSP garlic powder
2 tsps black pepper
2 tsps dried hot pepper, crushed
1 tsp ginger, ground
8 pieces chicken, skinless (4 breasts, 4 drumsticks)
1 tsp vegetable oil (use to grease baking pan)
a few shakes paprika

Directions

1. Preheat oven to 350 degrees F.
2. Add 1/2 teaspoon of poultry seasoning to milk.
3. Combine all other spices with cornflake crumbs and place in a plastic bag.
4. Wash chicken and pat dry. Dip chicken into milk, shake to remove excess, then quickly shake in bag with seasoning and crumbs.
5. Refrigerate for 1 hour.
6. Remove from refrigerator and sprinkle lightly with paprika for color.
7. Evenly space the chicken pieces on a greased baking pan.
8. Cover with aluminum foil and bake for 40 minutes.
9. Remove foil and continue baking for an additional 30 to 40 minutes or until the meat can be easily pulled away from the bone with a fork. The drumsticks may require less baking time than the breasts. Crumbs will form a crispy "skin." (Do not turn chicken during baking.)

Nutritional information (per serving): Calories 256, Sodium 286mg

Baked Chicken and Wild Rice

There are many low-fat versions of chicken and rice, and we particularly like this one because we use the spices tarragon and ginger mixed with white wine to nicely add the needed flavor to the sodium free chicken broth*. We avoid extra fat in this recipe by gently poaching the chicken and vegetables in the broth before baking it in the oven. Both white and wild rice are included and generous portions of sliced fresh mushrooms and chopped celery complete the dish. This is not only a perfect meal for those with acid reflux, but it is also great for family meals and small gatherings. Enjoy!

Recipe serves 4

Ingredients

1 pound white chicken breast meat cut into 1/2 to 1 inch pieces
1 cup chopped celery
1/2 cup sliced fresh mushrooms
2 cups sodium free chicken broth
1 1/2 cups white wine
3/4 cup uncooked white rice
3/4 cup uncooked wild rice
1 tsp fresh tarragon (or dried)
1 tsp organic chopped ginger (or ground)

Directions

1. Pour 1 cup of chicken broth into a large nonstick pot. Add the chicken, mushrooms, celery and spices. Bring to a simmer and cook for about 8 minutes or until chicken and veggies are tender.
2. Let the mixture cool
3. Pour the rice into a baking dish and add the wine and remaining chicken broth. Let it soak for 30 minutes.
4. Preheat the oven to 325 degrees.
5. Add the chicken and vegetable mixture to the baking dish and stir well.
6. Bake for 60 minutes, checking at 45 minutes to make sure the rice is not getting dry, and if it looks dry, add more chicken broth.

Nutritional information: Calories 330, Sodium 180mg

*We used Herb Ox sodium free chicken bouillon, which contains 0 g sodium and 10 calories per teaspoon. In comparison, regular chicken bouillon is 680 g sodium and 38 calories per teaspoon.

Healthy Pot Pie

Pot pies are great when the weather turns cold – they're warm and comforting for winter. But they are not the healthiest of meals. This recipe is a spin on a traditional pot pie that is much healthier. It uses lower fat ingredients, low fat and low cholesterol meats, and incorporates veggies to fill you up. It also uses whole wheat flour in the crust to give you more fiber. This pot pie is quick and easy to make and is a great way to use up leftovers. And you can always use a store-bought crust if you want to save time.

Recipe serves 8

Ingredients

For the crust

1 cup whole wheat flour
1 cup all purpose flour
½ tsp salt
6 TBSP water
1 cup butter spread (like smart balance or earth balance)

For the filling

3 cups shredded or chopped turkey or chicken
2 cups chopped potatoes
1 cup no salt added frozen mixed vegetables
(usually peas, carrots, and corn. Asparagus is great, too!)
1/3 cup green onions or leeks
1/3 cup chopped celery
1/3 cup butter spread
2/3 cups milk
1 cup low sodium chicken stock
1/3 cup all purpose flour
½ tsp salt and pepper mixed together

Directions

1. Preheat the oven to 425 degrees.
2. Mix the flour and salt for the crust into a bowl
3. Using a pastry blender or knife "cut in" the cup of butter spread.
4. Continue cutting in until the mixture looks like coarse crumbs or cornmeal.
5. Then begin slowly sprinkling the water over the dough 1-1/2 tsp at a time, using a fork fold the dough over in the water and mix. Another 1 TBSP of water may be needed if the dough is too dry.
6. Once all the water is added shape the dough into a ball and refrigerate for 30 minutes.
7. While dough is chilling, place the butter spread for filling in a pan and sauté the celery and leeks/ green onions until tender. Then add the 1/3 cup flour, salt, and pepper.
8. Stir in the broth and then the milk, stirring constantly until broth thickens.
9. Then add the meat, potatoes, and mixed veggies. Turn the heat off.

10. Remove the dough from the fridge and split in half.
11. Place each half flattened between two pieces of wax paper and roll out the dough until it is about 1/8 of an inch thick.
12. Place one half of dough in the 9" pie pan.
13. Place filling in the pie pan.
14. Cover filling and bottom crust with the top half of the crust.
15. Using a knife cut a couple of slits in the top of the dough to allow steam to escape.
16. Bake 30-40 minutes until the crust is brown and the potatoes are soft.
17. Let the pie stand for 5 minutes to cool and thicken before cutting.
18. ENJOY!

Nutritional information (per serving): Calories 327, Sodium 800mg

Enchiladas Verde

This take on traditional Mexican food is lightened up and adapted for people with acid reflux, so you can enjoy the flavor of Mexican food without the pain. Instead of a traditional red sauce, this recipe uses a Verde, or green, sauce made from tomatillos. It's light on the heat, but still gives the satisfying taste of Mexican food without the pain later. While tomatillos look like green tomatoes, they aren't actually tomatoes and shouldn't bother most people with acid reflux. You'll also notice that this recipe includes peppers. While they trigger symptoms on some people, they actually have anti-inflammatory properties, so there's not need to avoid them if they don't bother you. If you like some spice, keep the seeds in the peppers. If you do not like it at all, remove them. Don't forget the yogurt added to the sauce will reduce the heat, as well. Of course, everyone has different triggers, so you should avoid the tomatillos or peppers if you find they are a trigger for you.

Recipe serves 8 (2 enchiladas per serving)

Ingredients

6 chicken thighs
1 pound fresh (husks removed) or canned tomatillos, quartered
2 TBSP sage
3 cloves garlic
1/8 tsp salt
1/8 tsp pepper
1 bunch cilantro
16 corn tortillas
¼ cup non-fat Greek yogurt
1/8 cup canola oil
2 jalapenos or Serrano peppers, chopped
4 oz. Queso fresco or shredded Mexican cheese

Directions

1. Place chicken thighs in a pot and cover with about 2 cups of water. Add garlic, salt, pepper and cook on medium heat until chicken is cooked through (about 20 minutes).
2. Remove the chicken from the pot and place quartered tomatillos and chopped peppers in the water. Cook over medium heat until the tomatillos are heated and turn a brighter green.
3. While the tomatillos cook, remove the skin from the chicken and shred the chicken off the bones.
4. Once the tomatillos are heated, transfer the mixture from the pot to a blender. Add

the sage, cilantro and yogurt and blend until smooth.

5. In a small pan heat just enough canola oil to cover bottom of the pan. Place the tortillas in the pan one at a time and heat evenly on each side.

6. Add a portion of the chicken and sauce to each tortilla and then roll the tortilla. Remember to portion the chicken so you can fill 16 tortillas. Save most of the sauce to cover the tops of the enchiladas.

7. Place each rolled enchilada in a baking pan with the seam of the tortilla facing down to prevent them from unrolling.

8. Cover the rolled enchiladas with the remaining sauce and spread shredded cheese evenly over the tops.

9. Bake at 350 degrees for about 15 minutes until the cheese is melted and the enchiladas and sauce are warmed through.

Nutritional information (per serving): Calories 245, Sodium 149 mg

Chicken and Mushroom Cheese Bake

When fall approaches, our thoughts trend away from the barbecue and we start to think about "comfort foods." This baked casserole recipe is a family favorite! It uses low-fat ingredients like skim milk and reduced fat cheese to make it heartburn friendly. Add a healthy dose of steamed broccoli for a perfect side dish.

Recipe serves 4-6

Ingredients

5 slices whole wheat bread
5 tsp low fat margarine
4 skinless and boneless chicken breasts
1 4-ounce can of mushrooms, well drained
6 eggs
1 1/2 cups of reduced fat cheddar
1 1/2 cups skim milk
Pinch of salt (optional)

Directions

1. Preheat your oven to 350 degrees.
2. Cook chicken and cut into small cubes.
3. Cut crusts off bread and cube them.
4. Lightly spread margarine on both sides of the bread.
5. Cut each slice of bread diagonally into triangles and stand them around the edges of a 9 x 13 inch baking dish.
6. Spread the cubed pieces of the crust around the bottom of the dish.
7. Spread the cubed chicken and cheese over the bread cubes.
8. Combine the milk, eggs, and salt in a small bowl and whisk. Pour the mixture over the chicken and place the mushrooms on top.
9. Bake uncovered for 40 to 50 minutes until eggs look set and top is golden and puffy.

Nutritional information (per serving): Calories 365, Sodium 240mg

Curry Almond Chicken

This is a nice, light summer dish. We usually pair this with dark green veggies, and since the curry gives the chicken a yellow color, it makes a fun, colorful plate. Curry is often a misunderstood seasoning. Many mild curries can add a great amount of flavor to a dish without irritating GERD like spicy flavors can. In addition, curry powder is made with turmeric, which contains a powerful antioxidant. Interestingly, some research suggests that turmeric has anti-cancer properties that could be beneficial to GERD patients who are more susceptible to Barrett's Esophagus.

This recipe is packed with protein from the chicken and almond milk, but removing the skin from the chicken keeps the fat content low. And the almond milk adds a healthy dose of calcium. Enjoy!

Recipe serves 6

Ingredients

12 boneless skinless chicken thighs
2 cloves garlic
1 cup almond milk
1 TBSP olive oil
½ tsp nutmeg
1 tsp curry
1 bay leaf
1 cup chicken stock
½ cup sliced almonds

Directions

1. Preheat the oven to 400 degrees.
2. Chop garlic cloves and place in oven-safe pan with 1 teaspoon olive oil. Heat over medium-low heat and let cook for 3-4 minutes.
3. In a separate small pan toast the almonds with a touch of olive oil and set aside.
4. Once the garlic is browned, add the chicken thighs, almond milk, curry, nutmeg, chicken stock, and the bay leaf.
5. Let simmer on medium-low for 25 minutes.
6. Place pan in the oven for 20 minutes.
7. To serve, top the chicken with the toasted almonds.

Nutritional information (per serving): Calories 249, Sodium 252mg

Slow cooker Sunday supper

What's better than spending a Sunday afternoon surrounded by the wonderful aromas of your kitchen, or better yet spending a nice day out, and coming home with dinner ready to serve? This recipe is a cinch to make in your slow cooker and it's a twist on the classic "Chicken Marbella" dish that calls for lots of garlic. The chicken pieces are cooked with brown sugar, prunes, capers and olives, which might sound like an odd combination, but it makes a lovely complexity of flavors. The liquid base is spiced up with GERD diet friendly herbs, and is delicious when poured over some healthy rice. If you don't like prunes, you can easily substitute dried apricots. This is a dinner that's hard to beat and perfect for a family Sunday.

Yields 6-8 servings

Ingredients

4 TBSP packed brown sugar
4 TBSP white wine
4 TBSP red wine vinegar (divided)
2 TBSP dried oregano
3 bay leaves
1 tsp celery salt
1/2 tsp pepper
2 TBSP capers with a bit of juice
1/2 cup large pitted Spanish green olives cut in half
1 cup prunes
8 small chicken legs bone in (about 4 pounds split with skin removed)
1/4 cup chopped fresh parsley or chopped cilantro

Directions

1. In a large slow cooker whisk together the brown sugar, oregano, wine, 2 TBSP of vinegar with 1/2 cup of water, and add salt and pepper.
2. Add bay leaves, capers, olives, and prunes, and stir well.
3. Place the chicken pieces in the pot and surround them with the olives and prunes.
4. Cover and cook on low for 5 to 6 hours or on high for 3 to 4 hours.
5. Thirty minutes before serving, gently mix in parsley or cilantro and remaining 2 TBSP vinegar.
6. Remove chicken when ready and place on a platter with prunes and olives.
7. Reserve liquid, heat, and pour into a sauce boat to serve over rice.

Nutritional information (per serving): Calories 220, Sodium 385mg

Stuffed Turkey Rolls "Cordon Bleu"

This stuffed and rolled dish is fun to make, so put on your creative hat and give it a try. It takes a little effort, but we guarantee it is worth the time. The turkey rolls will look yummy on your plate, so both your company and your family will be impressed! We consider this recipe a low calorie version of "cordon bleu", one of the ultimate comfort foods! We kept it lower in fat and sodium by using low fat Swiss cheese and low sodium (but delicious!) smoked ham for the filling. We omitted salt and did a light sprinkle of pepper on each cutlet, and ramped up the flavor by mixing thyme and ginger into the breadcrumbs. These two spices are considered GERD friendly, so enjoy!

Makes 4 servings

Ingredients

4 1/4 pound turkey breast cutlets
1/2 tsp black pepper
4 (1 ounce) slices smoked ham, low fat, low sodium
2 (1 ounce) reduced fat Swiss cheese slices
3 TBSP plain dry breadcrumbs
1 teaspoon dried thyme
1/2 tsp ground ginger
1 TBSP low fat mayonnaise
1/4 cup dry white wine
1/4 low-sodium chicken broth
1 TBSP soft margarine

Directions

1. Season the cutlets with pepper and place 1 slice of ham and 1/2 slice of cheese on top of each piece of the turkey. Roll up and secure with toothpicks.
2. Mix the breadcrumbs with ginger and thyme.
3. Brush the rolled up cutlets with the mayonnaise and coat with the breadcrumb mixture. Pack them lightly so they adhere.
4. Spray a large skillet with nonstick cooking spray , and bring to medium heat. Add the rolls and cook until golden brown on all sides, about 4 to 5 minutes.
5. Add the wine, margarine, and chicken broth and bring to a boil. Cover the pan and reduce heat to a simmer.
6. Cook about five minutes longer until the turkey is thoroughly cooked and the sauce thickens.

Nutritional information (for 1 turkey roll): Calories 146, Sodium 420mg

Turkey Stroganoff

This hearty comfort dish has a long history, having originated in 19th century Russia and named for a prominent member of the "Stroganoff" family. For our GERD diet friendly stroganoff, we use a turkey breast, and slow cook it with fresh carrots and mushrooms. We then add peas and swirl in a mixture of Marsala wine, sour cream, and mustard. The alcohol in the wine should cook off, so it shouldn't trigger symptoms, but you can substitute an equal amount of chicken broth for the sauce if you'd like. This dish is perfect to serve over noodles, and so delicious!

Makes 6 servings (1-1/4 cup stew and 1 cup noodles)

Ingredients
One 3 to 4 pound split turkey breast
1-1/2 pounds assorted mushrooms
3 large carrots, sliced
1 cup reduced fat sour cream
1/3 cup all purpose flour
1/4 cup Marsala wine or sherry
1 cup frozen peas (thawed and drained)
1 tsp salt
1/2 tsp pepper
1 tsp Dijon mustard
8 ounces whole wheat egg noodles
1/4 cup finely chopped parsley or dill

Directions
1. Put carrots and mushrooms into a 5 to 6 quart slow cooker.
2. Top with turkey (meat size down).
3. Cover and cook on high for 4 hours (low for 8 hours).
4. Remove the turkey and place on a cutting board.
5. In a medium size bowl, whisk together the sour cream, flour, wine, and mustard and pour into the slow cooker along with the peas, salt, and pepper. Stir well.
6. Cover and cook on high until the sauce thickens for about 15 to 20 minutes.
7. Cook noodles according to package directions and keep warm.
8. Remove the turkey meat from the bone and cut into bite size pieces. When ready to serve, stir the turkey pieces back into the sauce.
9. Serve over cooked noodles, sprinkled with parsley or dill.

Nutritional information (per serving): Calories 420, Sodium 548mg

Mustard Pork Loin with Cauliflower Puree

The cauliflower in this recipe is a great, healthy replacement for a starch; it has texture and fills you up like mashed potatoes, but is much lower in calories. It tastes great, too! The pork loin is a low fat cut of pork and generally has less saturated fat than red meat. This is a great dish if your husband is a meat and potatoes type or you want to trick your kids into eating vegetables. This is also a great spin on comfort food for a cold day.

Recipe serves 4

Ingredients

For the pork loin

2-3 pound pork loin (usually a ¼ pound per person is adequate)

1 package leek soup mix (dry)

Dijon mustard

For the whipped cauliflower

1 head of cauliflower

½ cup of milk

2 garlic or shallot cloves

Shredded Monterey Jack cheese

¼ cup parsley chopped

Directions

1. Preheat the oven to 350 degrees.
2. Cover the outside of the pork with a thin layer of mustard, and then sprinkle the soup mix on the mustard.
3. Cook in the oven for about one hour or until the center is no longer pink and is 145⁰ internally.
4. While the pork loin is roasting, cut the cauliflower into large pieces.
5. Place the cauliflower and garlic in a steamer basket and steam for 10-15 minutes or until cauliflower breaks apart easily with a fork.
6. Once tender, place the cauliflower, garlic, and milk in the blender and puree.
7. Place puree back in the empty pot (water has been drained) and stir.
8. Add salt and pepper to taste.
9. Place each serving on a plate with a sprinkle of cheese and parsley.
10. Slice the pork loin and serve.

Nutritional Information (Per Serving):

Cauliflower Puree: Calories 93, Sodium 130mg

Pork Loin: Calories 215, Sodium 430mg

Whole Wheat Empanadas

We adapted this recipe to increase the amount of fiber and reduce the amount of fat to make the empanadas easier to digest for people with reflux disease. These empanadas are very filling because a quarter of the calories come from protein and they are much higher in fiber than white flour empanadas. To reduce the amount of fat in the recipe, we used a mixture of smart balance and olive oil instead of butter in the dough and used no added fat in the filling. Empanadas are traditionally fried, so baking them instead also reduces the amount of fat significantly. These empanadas can be prepared ahead and then heated to take on the go, for a snack, or in your child's lunch. They even freeze well. This is a fun, different dish and very filling for the amount of calories!

Recipe serves 10

Ingredients

For the dough

6 TBSP Smart Balance or other butter substitute spread

1 ½ TBSP Olive Oil

1 TBSP White Vinegar

1 cup Water

1/2 tsp Salt

3 cup Whole Wheat Flour

For the filling

1 pound ground turkey

1 tsp Garlic Powder

1/2 tsp paprika

1 tsp Taco seasoning

½ TBSP Worcestershire

8 oz Mushrooms chopped

Spinach – Frozen Chopped, defrosted and water squeezed out

Directions

1. Mix all of the ingredients for the dough except the whole wheat flour in a sauce pan. Heat until they come to a boil. Remove from heat.
2. Put flour in a bowl and add warm ingredients. Stir until smooth using a spatula.
3. Knead until dough is firm. If dough appears too watery or dry add a 1 TBSP of either water or flour to compensate.
4. Divide into 10 medium sized disks and freeze at least 2 hours. The dough can be prepared a day in advance if this is more convenient and freeze until ready to thaw the next day.
5. After 2 hours remove shells from freezer to defrost.
6. To prepare filling, cook ground turkey over medium-high heat until browned with no pink raw meat visible. Keep breaking apart turkey into small pieces.
7. Add the chopped mushrooms, spinach, and seasonings to the turkey and cook until all liquid has evaporated. Remove from heat.
8. Roll the dough into circles about 8" in diameter. The dough should be about ⅛" - ¼" inch thick. Do not add more flour when rolling because it will take away from

the adhesiveness of the dough and they will not fold or seal easily.

9. Fill empanadas by placing about 2-3 oz. of filling in the middle of each circle. Make sure there is enough room to fold them.
10. Softly fold the empanadas and use a fork seal the edges into a half circle.
11. Bake at 350 degrees for 8-10 minutes until light brown. The color will be lighter than the unbaked dough.

Nutritional information (per serving): Calories 260, Sodium 525mg

Stuffed pork tenderloin

Any recipe that calls for "stuffing" gets our attention, and our lightened up microwaveable version of this classic pork dish is delicious. It's quick and easy and should not trigger your heartburn symptoms. Simply mix together the stuffing ingredients, place them in a glass dish and gently top the mixture with the pork tenderloins and chicken soup. And then voila, dinner will be ready in just minutes! Keep in mind that for safe microwaving, you will need to carefully follow the cooking instructions. Enjoy!

Yields 4 servings

Ingredients

6 slices reduced fat white bread, toasted and cubed
1/2 cup finely chopped cauliflower
1 cup finely chopped celery
3/4 cup water
1 tsp poultry seasoning
1 tsp dried parsley flakes
4 (3.5 to 4 oz tenderized) pork tenderloins
1 can reduced fat cream of chicken soup

Directions

1. In a large bowl, combine bread cubes, cauliflower, and celery. Add water, poultry seasoning, and parsley. Stir gently to mix.
2. Distribute the mixture evenly in a 8 x 8 inch microwaveable glass baking dish and pat down.
3. Place the tenderloins evenly on top of the stuffing.
4. Spoon chicken soup evenly over the top.
5. Cover with plastic wrap making sure it will not touch the food during cooking, and cut 2 one inch vents to let the steam escape.
6. Microwave on high (100 percent power) for 15 minutes and turn*, then continue to cook another 10 minutes until pork is tender.
7. Let this dish set for 3 minutes and divide into four serving.

*If your microwave has a rotating dish, there is no need to turn the dish

Nutritional information (per serving): Calories 283, Sodium 549mg

Easy Beef (or Pork) Burgundy

There are times when only beef can satisfy your taste buds and this classic dish does the trick for me! Since beef is more difficult to digest than other foods, we suggest that you use only lean beef, limit the frequency of beef in your meals, and keep the portion size small. For this recipe we recommend that you use beef tenderloin, a leaner cut of meat. For an interesting twist and a lower fat version, follow the same directions but substitute the same size pork tenderloin for the beef tenderloin! Remember to limit the meat portion to a healthy 3.5 oz and fill up on the veggies. And don't worry about the red wine - the alcohol will evaporate during cooking. As we say at our house...mmm mmm good!

Serves 4

Ingredients

1 pound beef tenderloin cut into 1 inch cubes
1/4 tsp black pepper
1/4 tsp salt
1 (12 ounce) package frozen vegetables with broccoli, carrots and cauliflower
1 (10 ounce) package of mushrooms
1 tsp dried thyme
2/3 cup burgundy or another dry red wine
1 cup reduced sodium fat free gravy

Directions

1. Sprinkle the beef with salt and pepper.
2. Spray the bottom of a Dutch oven with smart balance and heat to medium.
3. Add the beef and cook on all sides until brown, about 2 minutes.
4. Add the mushrooms, frozen vegetables, and thyme. Cook and stir for another minute.
5. Add the wine and bring to a boil. Reduce the heat and simmer for two minutes.
6. Add the gravy to the mixture and again bring it to a boil.
7. Reduce the heat and simmer until the mushrooms are fully cooked and the sauce thickens, about 4 more minutes.

Nutritional Information (per serving): Calories 233, Sodium 310mg

Gingersnap beef stew with red cabbage

Gingersnaps, cabbage, and caraway seeds give this stew a delightful flavor. We slow cook this dish with "eye of the round" which is an 'extra lean' cut of meat. Bottom round roast steak, sirloin tip side steak, top sirloin steak, and bottom round roast steak are also in the "extra lean" category. Keep in mind that by choosing one of these cuts, we reduced the fat content in this GERD diet friendly recipe by about half. When in doubt, your butcher is a great source for helping you identify the extra lean cuts of meat. Enjoy!

Recipe makes 5 servings

Ingredients

1-1/4 lb extra lean beef cut into 1-inch pieces
1 TBSP vegetable oil
2 large celery stalks, thinly sliced
1 TBSP Dried minced onion (optional)
1-1/2 C water
3/4 tsp caraway seeds
1/2 tsp salt
1/8 tsp black pepper
1 bay leaf
1/4 cup of white vinegar
1 TBSP sugar
1/2 small head red cabbage, cut into 4 wedges
1/4 cup of crushed gingersnaps

Directions

1. Brown meat in oil in a heavy skillet. Remove meat and sauté celery in remaining oil until golden.
2. Return meat to skillet. Add water, dried onion, caraway seeds, salt, pepper, and bay leaf. Bring to a boil.
3. Reduce heat, cover, and simmer 1-1/4 hours.
4. Add vinegar and sugar; stir. Place cabbage on top of meat. Cover and simmer 45 minutes more.
5. Arrange meat and cabbage on a platter and keep warm. Strain drippings and skim off fat.
6. Add enough water to drippings to yield 1 cup of liquid. Return to skillet with gingersnap crumbs.
7. Cook and stir until thickened and mixture boils. Serve with meat and vegetables.

Nutritional information (per serving): Calories: 244, Sodium 323mg

Beef and mushroom skillet

There are times when only beef will satisfy your taste buds, and this hearty skillet recipe will do the trick! We used a lean cut of meat (top round) and plain low-fat yogurt to keep the dish low in fat and GERD diet friendly. We flavored the sauce with nutmeg, ginger, and dried basil - all heartburn friendly spices. Be sure to limit your beef portion to a 3.5 oz serving and enjoy your favorite vegetables or some crusty bread on the side.

Yields 5 servings--Serving Size: 6 oz

Ingredients

1 pound lean beef (top round)
3 TBSP apple cider vinegar
2 tsp vegetable oil
3/4 TBSP dried minced onion*
1 pound sliced mushrooms
1/4 tsp salt
Pepper to taste
1/4 tsp nutmeg
1/4 tsp ginger
1/2 tsp dried basil
1/4 cup white wine
1 cup plain low-fat yogurt
6 cup cooked macaroni, cooked in unsalted water

Directions

1. Cut beef into 1-inch cubes, and marinate for at least 2 hours in vinegar.
2. Heat 1 teaspoon oil in a non-stick skillet.
3. Add beef and sauté for 5 minutes. Turn to brown evenly. Remove from pan and keep hot.
4. Add remaining oil to pan; sauté mushrooms.
5. Add beef to pan with seasonings.
6. Add wine, yogurt, and dried onion; gently stir in. Heat, but do not boil.
7. Serve with whole wheat pasta or brown rice

Note: If thickening is desired, use 2 teaspoons of cornstarch.

Nutritional Information (per serving): Calories 499, Sodium 200mg

*Omit onions if the dried form triggers your GERD symptoms.

Braised Short Ribs

Fall-off-the-bone ribs. Sounds delicious, doesn't it? This classic dish is perfect for the slow cooker on a cold winter day. And paired with lots of veggies, this dish packs a nutritional punch. The broth is loaded with vitamins and minerals from cooking the bones, herbs, and veggies. This recipe includes beer, but the alcohol evaporates in the cooking process, so it shouldn't affect your GERD symptoms. One other thing to note - it's recommended to limit red meat when you have GERD because of the high fat content. This recipe as prepared only has 9 grams of fat per serving because the fat cooks off as you braise the ribs and ends up in the liquid. Be sure to use a slotted spoon when serving this dish to leave the fat in the pot.

The dish is quick to put together, but it does take a few hours to slow cook. You can just leave it on the burner or in the slow cooker while you go about your day. Enjoy!

Recipe serves 4

Ingredients

3 pounds short ribs, bone in (approximately 8 ribs, 2 per person)
½ cup flour
1 12 oz bottle pale ale
4 beef bouillon cubes
1 parsnip
2 carrots
½ shallot
3 cloves garlic
1 tsp rosemary
2 tsp thyme
2 bay leaves

Directions

1. Salt and pepper the short ribs.
2. Heat a large skillet over medium-high heat.
3. Place four in a large bowl and coat each short rib thoroughly in the flour.
4. Place the ribs in the skillet so all of one side is touching skillet. Set a timer for 5 minutes, and do not touch or turn ribs until timer has gone off.
5. Once the timer goes off, turn the ribs to the other side and let sear 5 more minutes. They should appear dark brown on the outside once done.
6. While the ribs are searing, pour the pale ale into the slow cooker and add the bouillon, bay leaves, thyme and rosemary. Set the slow cooker on high. If you're cooking these on the stovetop, add the same ingredients to a large pot and turn on low heat.

7. Chop the garlic and shallot, and dice the parsnip and carrots as the ribs finish cooking.
8. Place the ribs in the pot/slow cooker. Do not drain fat from the skillet.
9. Place vegetables in the skillet let the beef fat cook the vegetables until shallots are translucent and carrots and parsnips soften and brown (approximately 5-10 minutes).
10. Add the vegetables to pot. Let cook for 3 hours and enjoy. You will have perfect fall-off-the-bone short ribs!
11. To serve, use a slotted spoon to place some of the vegetables on each plate then top with two ribs.

Nutritional information (for 2 ribs & ¼ cup vegetables): Calories 165, Sodium 330mg

Oven steamed tilapia

This recipe is delicious, healthy, and very fast to make – perfect for a busy weeknight!

Some people with reflux disease avoid fish dishes because they are often paired with citrus – lemon and lime – which can cause their reflux symptoms to flare up. But this recipe is actually stomach settling, thanks to the ginger.

It pairs nicely with an Asian vegetable, like bok choy or sautéed snow peas, and brown rice. Remember, though, that rice takes a lot longer to cook than this dish, so plan ahead. Whatever it is served with, steaming the fish in parchment paper cooks it perfectly!

The following directions are for one serving of fish. Plan for one filet per person and repeat this process for each one.

Ingredients

3-4 oz tilapia Filet
1 tsp olive or canola oil
1 inch slices of fresh ginger to cover the fish
1 tsp low sodium soy sauce
1 dash paprika
1 dash garlic powder
1 sheet of parchment paper large enough to wrap the fish

Directions

1. Place fish in the center of the parchment paper.
2. Sprinkle the fish with paprika and garlic powder.
3. Pour olive oil and soy sauce on top.
4. Place thinly sliced ginger on top of fish covering most of fish.
5. Fold parchment paper by pulling each of the four corners into the center and folding edges carefully to seal. Place packets on a baking sheet.
6. Preheat oven to 350 degrees.
7. Cook 15-20 minutes. The fish is done when it is white (not opaque or pink) and flakes easily with a fork.

Nutritional information (per serving): Calories 159, Sodium 123mg

Shrimp and pea stir fry

Stir-fries are easy to create and are perfect for busy nights when you are pressed for time. Because stir frying is fast, you will want to have the ingredients prepped and ready to go before you start cooking. For this GERD diet friendly entree, we use fresh shrimp, cabbage, sweet bell pepper, and frozen peas. The peas add an extra punch of fiber to the recipe and nutrient rich white cabbage provides a terrific crunch. We season the mixture with fresh ginger to give it a nice peppery zest, and serve it alone or over some brown rice or noodles. It's a meal that's good for your health and packed with flavor, too!

Yields 4 servings

Ingredients

1 fresh sweet bell pepper (chopped)
2 TBSP finely grated ginger
2/3 pound white cabbage (sliced into thin strips)
1 TBSP olive or canola oil
1 tsp sesame oil
1-1/2 cups frozen peas
3/4 pound cooked and peeled large shrimp
4 TBSP chopped fresh cilantro

Directions

1. Heat both oils to a high heat in a large frying pan.
2. Stir-fry the ginger and chopped bell pepper for 5 seconds and then add the peas.
3. Continue to stir-fry the mixture about 2 minutes until the peas are thawed.
4. Add the cabbage and stir-fry for an additional 2 to 3 minutes.
5. Add the shrimp and cook for approximately one minute to heat through.
6. Stir in the cilantro and serve immediately.

Nutritional information (per serving): Calories 185, Sodium 80mg

Roasted Salmon with Mango Honey Soy Glaze

This recipe is easy to prepare and so delicious even those who are not big salmon fans will love it. The healthy benefits include mango, which is rich in dietary fiber, and honey, which can help build up immunities (because local honey has pollen from your area). Salt and pepper and garlic are optional. For those who can tolerate scallions, put a few slices on top of the cooked fish and enjoy!

Recipe serves 4

Ingredients

1/4 cup of puréed ripe mango
1 1/2 tsp lower sodium soy sauce
1/2 tsp kosher salt (optional)
1/2 tsp ground pepper (optional)
1/8 tsp garlic (optional)
2 TBSP local honey
4 (6 ounce) salmon filets
Cooking spray

Directions

1. Preheat your oven to 450 degrees.
2. Combine crushed ripe mango, soy sauce and honey (salt and pepper and garlic are optional) in a small bowl. Arrange salmon filets on a foil lined baking sheet coated with cooking spray. Brush fillets evenly with half of the marinade mixture. Bake salmon at 450 for 4 minutes.
3. Heat broiler to high. Do not open the oven or remove the salmon. Broil fish for 6 more minutes.
4. Open oven and spoon remaining mixture onto the center of the fish fillets. Continue to broil the fish an additional 3 minutes.
5. Carefully remove the salmon from the oven and let sit for five minutes before serving. ENJOY!

Nutritional information (per serving): Calories 305, Sodium 425mg

Elegant dover sole

Dover sole is a mild white fish with a delicate buttery flavor. It is also a "flat" firm fish, which makes it ideal for stuffing and rolling. This recipe is made with spinach and mushrooms, and seasoned with oregano to give it a Mediterranean flair. We use just a scant amount of oil, and part-skim mozzarella cheese to keep the dish low in fat and GERD diet friendly. A dash of garlic powder is optional and should be omitted if the dried herb triggers your heartburn symptoms. Buon appetito!

Makes 4 servings (serving size: 1 fillet roll)

Ingredients
1 tsp olive oil
1/2 pound fresh mushrooms, sliced
1/2 pound fresh spinach, chopped
1/4 tsp dried oregano
1/4 tsp garlic powder*
1/8 tsp pepper
1-1/2 pounds Dover sole fillets
2 TBSP sherry
4 oz part-skim mozzarella cheese, grated

Directions
1. Preheat oven to 400 degrees F.
2. Spray a 10x6-inch baking dish with nonstick cooking spray.
3. Heat oil in skillet; sauté mushrooms about 3 minutes or until tender.
4. Add spinach and continue cooking about 1 minute or until spinach is barely wilted.
5. Remove from heat; drain liquid into prepared baking dish.
6. Add oregano and garlic to drained vegetables; stir to mix ingredients.
7. Divide vegetable mixture evenly among fillets, placing filling in center of each fillet.
8. Roll fillet around mixture and place seam-side down in prepared baking dish.
9. Sprinkle with sherry, then grated mozzarella cheese. Bake 15-20 minutes or until fish flakes easily. Lift out with a slotted spoon.

Nutritional information (per serving): Calories 262, Sodium 312mg

Fish fillets in parchment

Cooking "en papilotte," or in parchment paper, is incredibly easy and a great way to prepare delicious GERD diet friendly meals. For this fish recipe, the fillets are steamed with vegetables in individual parchment packets. This allows the juices to blend, retaining the flavor of each ingredient. The packets are ideal for a single serving when you are cooking for one, and can be put together a day in advance for convenience. Clean up is a snap too as you simply crumple up the paper and throw it away. This cooking technique is foolproof even for rookies, but a couple of guidelines are important. Number one: be sure to carefully close the packets so that steam does not escape, and two: never open the packets while cooking! Enjoy!

Recipe makes 1 serving

Ingredients

4 ounce white fish fillets (snapper, cod, or halibut)
1/4 cup chopped fresh broccoli
1 small red potato chopped
1/4 cup julienne cut carrot
1 TBSP whole capers
A few herbs such as ginger, thyme, basil, parsley, or cilantro
Olive oil (about 1 TBSP)
Black pepper

Directions

1. Preheat oven to 450 degrees.
2. Make a 14 inch square of parchment paper.
3. Fold over to make a triangle and place fish in the center of the fold.
4. Top with all ingredients.
5. Sprinkle with herbs and pepper and drizzle with olive oil.
6. Crimp edges over to make a seal and twist the ends up to secure tightly.
7. Place packet on baking sheet and bake for 15 minutes.
8. Carefully cut open and serve immediately.

Nutritional information (per serving): Calories 310, Sodium 171mg

Grilled Caesar Swordfish

Swordfish is a very popular and healthy fish. It is low in calories, but high in protein and has a consistency that makes it perfect the grill! We first marinate the fish in a reduced fat Caesar salad dressing for 30 minutes. This gives the fish a unique flavor that pairs nicely with the romaine lettuce leaves. The ingredients are low in fat and GERD friendly, but if you can tolerate a splash of lemon, go for it! Serve with grilled vegetables tossed with a dash of balsamic vinegar to round out the meal. Bon appetit!

Makes 6 servings

Ingredients

2 pounds fresh swordfish steaks
1/3 cup reduced fat Caesar salad dressing
20 small romaine lettuce leaves
2 TBSP crushed plain croutons
2 TBSP extra virgin olive oil
1 TBSP grated Parmesan cheese
Black pepper (optional)
Splash of lemon (optional)

Directions

1. Pour the salad dressing over the fish and marinade for 1 hour in the refrigerator.
2. Turn the fish over once after 30 minutes (halfway).
3. Coat the grill with non-stick cooking spray and heat the grill to medium.
4. Place the fish on the grill rack about 4 to 5 inches above the heat.
5. Cook the fish about 5 minutes and flip over. Continue cooking until the fish flakes nicely with a fork (about 4 more minutes). Remove from grill, cover with foil, and let rest for 2 minutes.
6. Tear the lettuce leaves into pieces and toss in large bowl with the olive oil. Sprinkle the leaves with Parmesan cheese and crushed croutons. Mix well and divide equally onto six plates.
7. Cut the fish into 6 equal portions and place on top of the prepared lettuce leaves.
8. Lightly sprinkle each plate with black pepper, if desired.

Nutritional information: Calories 302, Sodium 295mg

White Fish Veronica

Seasoned fresh white fish, a dash of lemon, and lots of seedless grapes combine to make a delectable and healthy GERD diet friendly entree. Low-sodium chicken broth and low-fat milk reduce the fat content for this recipe, yet still give the sauce a rich creamy taste. Choose one of the fish types listed below, and use the freshest one available at your market. I like to serve this fish dish on a bed of sautéed spinach, because it is so very healthy...and tasty too!

Makes 4 servings

Ingredients

1 pound white fish (cod, sole, turbot, orange roughy, tilapia)
1/4 tsp salt
1/8 tsp black pepper
1/4 cup of dry white wine
1/4 cup of low-sodium chicken broth, skim fat from top
1 TBSP lemon juice*
1 TBSP soft margarine
2 TBSP flour
3/4 cup of low-fat (1%) or skim milk
1 cup of seedless grapes
Non stick cooking spray as needed

Directions

1. Spray 10x6-inch baking dish with nonstick spray.
2. Place fish in pan and sprinkle with salt and pepper.
3. Mix wine, stock, and lemon juice in small bowl and pour over fish.
4. Cover and bake at 350 degrees F for 15 minutes.
5. Melt margarine in small saucepan.
6. Remove from heat and blend in flour. Gradually add milk and cook over moderately low heat, stirring constantly until thickened.
7. Remove fish from oven and pour liquid from baking dish into cream sauce, stirring until blended.
8. Pour sauce over fish and sprinkle with grapes.
9. Broil about 4 inches from heat 5 minutes or until sauce starts to brown.

*If a small amount of lemon triggers your heartburn symptoms, omit or substitute with apple cider vinegar, if desired.

Nutritional information (per serving): Calories: 148, Sodium 316mg

Trout almondine

For this GERD diet friendly entree, we broil fresh trout fillets in a flavorful basil and ginger infused olive oil. Sliced bell peppers and almonds complete the dish, and we like to serve brown rice on the side. It's a quick and easy dinner recipe for weeknights, but also nice enough for special occasions. Moist and tender, the fillets are virtually fat free and will melt in your mouth. It's a "guilt-free" meal and delicious too!

Recipe serves 4

Ingredients

1-1/4 TBSP olive oil
1/2 tsp dried basil
1/2 tsp ground ginger
4 trout fillets
2 large red, yellow or green bell peppers
1/3 cup sliced unsalted almonds
4 lemon wedges (omit if it triggers your GERD symptoms)

Directions

1. Preheat the broiler to high.
2. Whisk oil and herbs together in a small bowl. Line a broiler pan with foil and brush lightly with the oil.
3. Arrange the fish fillets skin side down on foil in the center of the pan.
4. Slice the peppers into 1/2 inch slices and place them around the fish.
5. Brush the trout and peppers with prepared oil and broil for 2 to 3 minutes. Turn the fillets over and brush with more oil. Continue to broil for another 2 to 3 minutes until bubbling or beginning to crisp.
6. Carefully place almonds on top of the fish and broil for a minute or less until golden brown.
7. Transfer to plates and serve immediately.

Nutritional information (per serving): Calories 365, Sodium 35mg

Tuna casserole

There is nothing as reliably delicious as a traditional tuna casserole, but it is very fattening, so modifications are a must for people watching their weight. For this GERD diet friendly version, we use fat-free milk, low-fat plain yogurt, and reduced-fat cream of mushroom soup flavored with Dijon mustard and Italian herbs. Mmm Mmm! It adds up to delicious and surprisingly creamy. It reheats nicely too!

Yields 4 - 5 servings

Ingredients

1 (12 oz) package egg noodles
1 can tuna (7 oz in water)
1 cup frozen peas (thawed)
1 can (10-3/4 oz) reduced-fat cream of mushroom soup
1/4 cup fat-free plain yogurt
1/2 cup fat-free milk
1 TBSP Dijon mustard
1/4 tsp pepper
1/4 tsp dried basil
2 oz low-fat shredded cheddar
10 crushed "baked" potato chips
Fresh parsley

Directions

1. Boil noodles according to package directions.
2. Drain and flake tuna.
3. In a medium bowl, mix together soup, milk, yogurt, and mustard.
4. Stir in tuna and peas.
5. Place mixture into a 9-inch round baking dish, and gently stir in noodles.
6. Mix the cheese and chips together and sprinkle over the dish.
7. Bake at 350 degrees for 30 minutes.
8. If desired, sprinkle each serving with some fresh parsley.

Nutritional information (per 1 cup serving): Calories 261, Sodium 240mg

Healthy cornbread

Take a break from regular bread and try making this fluffy cornbread recipe. It's baked to perfection using 1% milk and a small amount of margarine to keep it lower in saturated fat and GERD diet friendly. The basic recipe is so easy and forgiving, you might find yourself making it often. For variety, you can add a teaspoon of heartburn friendly seasonings to the mixture - like cumin, ginger or cinnamon - or you can try folding in a 1/4 cup of fresh or canned corn, puréed beans, or grated cheese. Just add your selected ingredients, make a slight adjustment to the amount of liquid, as needed, and it's ready for the oven. Mmm Mmm good!

Makes 10 servings

Ingredients
1 cup cornmeal
1 cup flour
1/4 cup white sugar
1 tsp baking powder
1 cup buttermilk, 1% fat
1 egg, whole
1/4 cup margarine
1 tsp vegetable oil (to grease baking pan)

Directions
1. Preheat oven to 350 degrees F.
2. Mix together cornmeal, flour, sugar, and baking powder.
3. In another bowl, combine buttermilk and egg. Beat lightly.
4. Slowly add buttermilk and egg mixture to the dry ingredients.
5. Add margarine and mix by hand or with a mixer for 1 minute.
6. Bake for 20 to 25 minutes in a 8 by 8-inch greased baking dish. Cool.
7. Cut into 10 squares.

Nutritional information (per serving): Calories 178, Sodium 94mg

Homestyle southern biscuits

Biscuits have long been a staple of the American diet, especially in Southern states. Freshly baked early in the morning, breakfast biscuits are a tradition in the South and eaten with honey, butter, syrup, or jellies. They also make a perfect accompaniment for dinner soups and stews. We lightened up the old fashioned version to make them GERD diet friendly, so y'all enjoy! This recipe is finger lickin' good!

Makes 15 2-inch biscuits

Ingredients
2 cups flour
2 tsps baking powder
1/4 tsp baking soda
1/4 tsp salt
2 TBSP sugar
2/3 cup buttermilk, 1% fat
3 TBSP +1 tsp Vegetable oil

Directions

1. Preheat oven to 450 degrees F.
2. In a medium bowl, combine flour, baking powder, baking soda, salt, and sugar.
3. In a small bowl, stir together buttermilk and oil. Pour over flour mixture and stir until well mixed.
4. On a lightly floured surface, knead dough gently for 10 to 12 strokes.
5. Roll or pat dough to 3/4-inch thickness.
6. Cut with a 2-inch biscuit or cookie cutter, dipping cutter in flour between cuts.
7. Transfer biscuits to an ungreased baking sheet.
8. Bake for 12 minutes or until golden brown. Serve warm.

Nutritional information (per biscuit): Calories 99, Sodium 72mg

Savory Italian vegetables

Fresh vegetables can accompany a variety of main courses, and this quick and easy dish is one of our favorites. It's adapted from a friend's "tried and true" old family recipe that comes straight from Sicily. The original version calls for lemon instead of rice wine vinegar. The vinegar is a nice replacement - but if your GERD diet can tolerate a dash of lemon, go for it! And be sure to always choose the freshest available veggies for good health! As they say in Italy, Buon Appetito!

Makes four 1/2 cup servings

Ingredients

2 or 3 zucchini (sliced)
1 yellow squash (sliced)
1 Red bell pepper (diced)
1 tsp Marsala wine
1/4 tsp oregano
1/4 tsp brown sugar
1/4 tsp seasoned rice vinegar (or fresh lemon*)
1 tsp canola oil

Directions

1. Add canola oil to a large pan and heat to medium.
2. Add veggies and sauté for about two minutes, stirring often.
3. Add Marsala wine, brown sugar, oregano and vinegar.
4. Continue to cook until veggies are tender, but still slightly firm.

Nutritional information (per serving): Calories 29, Sodium 2mg

Sweet potato custard

For this recipe, we combine healthy sweet potatoes and bananas to make a flavorful GERD diet friendly custard-style dish. We kept the recipe lower in fat and cholesterol by using evaporated skim milk, and you can lighten it up even more by replacing the eggs yolks with your choice of egg substitute. It is flavored with cinnamon, a heartburn friendly spice, and nicely sweetened with some delicious raisins and brown sugar! This is a great side dish for holidays and dinner parties. It also pairs perfectly with just about anything, so give it a try!

Recipe makes 6 servings

Ingredients

1 cup mashed cooked sweet potato
1/2 cup mashed ripe banana (about 2 small)
1 cup evaporated skim milk
2 TBSP packed brown sugar
2 beaten egg yolks (or 1/3 cup egg substitute)
1/2 tsp salt
1/4 cup raisins
1 TBSP sugar
1 tsp ground cinnamon
Non-stick cooking spray as needed

Directions

1. In a medium bowl, stir together sweet potato and banana. Add milk, blending well.
2. Add brown sugar, egg yolks, and salt, mixing thoroughly.
3. Spray a 1-quart casserole with nonstick cooking spray. Transfer sweet potato mixture to casserole dish.
4. Combine raisins, sugar, and cinnamon; sprinkle over top of sweet potato mixture.
5. Bake in a preheated 325 degrees F oven for 40-45 minutes or until a knife inserted near center comes out clean.

Nutritional information (per serving): Calories 144, Sodium 235mg

Twice baked potatoes

This vegetable dish is delicious and made with GERD diet friendly ingredients, including the spices dill and ginger. The potatoes are twice baked and then stuffed, which requires a little extra time - but you will think it's worth the effort! It's a perfect side dish for a dinner party, and pairs well with meat, fish, or fowl. The recipe is a low fat, low-cholesterol and low-sodium treat, and can be made a day ahead for ease.

Makes 8 servings (1/2 potato per serving)

Ingredients

4 medium baking potatoes
3/4 cup of low-fat (1%) cottage cheese
1/4 cup of low-fat (1%) milk
2 TBSP soft margarine
1 tsp dill weed
1 tsp ginger
1/2 tsp pepper
2 tsp grated parmesan cheese

Directions

1. Wash potatoes and pierce the skin with a fork. Bake at 425 degrees F for 60 minutes or until fork is easily inserted.
2. Cut potatoes in half lengthwise. Carefully scoop out potato leaving about 1/2 inch of pulp inside shell.
3. Mash pulp in large bowl.
4. Mix in by hand remaining ingredients except parmesan cheese.
5. Spoon mixture into potato shells.
6. Sprinkle top with 1/4 tsp parmesan cheese.
7. Place on baking sheet and return to oven. Bake 15-20 minutes or until tops are golden brown.
8. If making a day ahead, do not sprinkle with cheese until ready to cook. Place cooled potatoes in an airtight container and refrigerate. Bake refrigerated potatoes for an extra 10 to 15 minutes.

Nutritional information (per serving): Calories 113, Sodium 136mg

Carolina potato pie

This "low country" inspired sweet potato pie is lightened up to make it GERD diet friendly. We use vegetable oil (instead of butter) and evaporated skim milk to do the trick. Sweet potatoes are loaded with healthy fiber, potassium, and vitamin A and have a few less calories than their white counterpart. This vegetable dish recipe is a delightful side for festive dinner parties, holidays and family meals, and pairs perfectly with pork, poultry, or beef. "In my mind I'm going to Carolina..."

Makes 16 servings

Ingredients

For the filling
1/4 cup white sugar
1/4 cup brown sugar
1/2 tsp salt
1/4 tsp nutmeg
3 large eggs, beaten
1/4 cup evaporated skim milk, canned
1 tsp vanilla extract
3 cups sweet potatoes (cooked and mashed)

For the crust
1 1/4 cups flour
1/4 tsp sugar
1/3 cup skim milk
2 TBSP vegetable oil

Directions

1. Preheat oven to 350 degrees F.
2. To make the crust, combine the flour and sugar in a bowl. Add milk and oil to the flour mixture, and stir with fork until well mixed and then form pastry into a smooth ball with your hands.
3. Roll the ball between two 12-inch squares of waxed paper using short, brisk strokes until pastry reaches edge of paper.
4. Peel off top paper and invert crust into pie plate.
5. For the filling, combine sugars, salt, spices, and eggs. Add milk and vanilla. Stir. Add sweet potatoes and mix well.
6. Pour mixture into pie shell.
7. Bake for 60 minutes or until crust is golden brown.
8. Cool and cut into 16 slices.

Nutritional information (per serving): Calories 147, Sodium 98mg

Baked French fries

Who doesn't love French fries? But fries without ketchup? We all know that tomato-based ketchup can trigger GERD symptoms, so we bake these fries in this recipe to extra crispy, which makes them perfect to dip in apple cider vinegar! If you have never tried fries dipped in vinegar, you are in for a treat. Oven baking makes these potatoes lower in fat that their fried cousins, which keeps this recipe GERD diet friendly. And remember, fries are best when they are crispy on the outside and creamy on the inside, so don't undercook!

Makes 5 servings--Serving size: 1 cup

Ingredients
4 large Russet or Idaho potatoes (2 lbs)
8 cups ice water
Apple cider vinegar
1 tsp garlic powder*
1 tsp onion powder*
1/4 tsp salt
1 tsp white pepper
1/4 tsp allspice
1 TBSP vegetable oil

Directions
1. Scrub potatoes and cut into long 1/2-inch strips.
2. Place potato strips into ice water, cover, and chill for 1 hour or longer.
3. Remove potatoes and dry strips thoroughly.
4. Place garlic powder, onion powder, salt, white pepper, allspice, and pepper flakes in a plastic bag.
5. Toss potatoes in spice mixture.
6. Brush potatoes with oil.
7. Place potatoes in nonstick shallow baking pan.
8. Cover with aluminum foil and place in 475 degrees F oven for 15 minutes.
9. Remove foil and continue baking uncovered for an additional 15 to 20 minutes or until golden brown and crispy!
10. Turn fries occasionally to brown on all sides.

Nutritional information (per serving): Calories 238, Sodium 163mg

*If the dried form of these herbs trigger your GERD symptoms, omit or substitute with your favorite GERD friendly spice.

Risotto with Parsley and Seasonal Vegetables

Topped with fresh, seasonal vegetables, this risotto is a colorful reminder of spring! The recipe uses seasonal vegetables, so you can choose between cauliflower and squash. If you do not like cauliflower, then yellow and green squash make good substitutes. Since it's loaded with vegetables, this dish is packed with fiber and vitamins. And the parsley makes the risotto bright green!

Recipe serves 10

Ingredients

2 cups Arborio rice
8 cups low-sodium chicken stock
4 cloves of garlic or 1 shallot
2 TBSP olive oil
½ cup white or red wine
2 bunches parsley
½ cup grated Parmesan cheese
¼ cup melted butter

2 bay leaves
1 tsp thyme
1 tsp rosemary
1 tsp salt
1 tsp black Pepper
2 heads cauliflower (Pick your color: green, white, purple, or yellow)
4 squash (Green and/or yellow)

Directions

1. In a large skillet combine olive oil and shallots/ garlic. Cook on medium heat until translucent (about 5 minutes).
2. Add risotto to the skillet and cook a few minutes.
3. Pour in the wine and stir the rice until the wine has entirely been absorbed.
4. Add salt pepper and bay leaves.
5. Add the chicken stock one cup at a time. Let all of the stock be absorbed by the rice before adding another cup. This step is crucial because if the stock is not absorbed, the rice will not get soft enough.
6. Once all the stock is absorbed, your rice grains should be larger, soft, and somewhat fluffy.
7. Using a blender or food processor, grind up the parsley along with a stick of butter.
8. Add the parsley/butter blend to the rice right before serving to maintain the bright green color.
9. Steam or sauté the cauliflower/squash (the colors will get much brighter) and place on top of and around the risotto.

Nutritional information (per serving): Calories 190, Sodium 202mg

Ginger pasta pilaf

This rice and pasta "pilaf" is low in fat and flavored with ginger, which makes it a perfect entree or side dish to include in your GERD diet plan. For this recipe, we first sauté the vermicelli with the onions - and then we minimize the fat content by draining the mixture well. You can substitute chopped celery for the onions* if sautéed onions trigger your heartburn symptoms. Serve this interesting mixture of pasta, rice, and vegetables alone or as a side for your favorite meat, chicken, or fish recipe. It's light, healthy, and delicious!

Yields 6 servings

Ingredients

2 TBSP olive oil
1/2 cup finely broken vermicelli, uncooked
2 TBSP chopped onions* or celery
1 cup long-grain white rice, uncooked
1-1/4 cup hot chicken stock (made with low sodium bouillon)
1-1/4 cup hot water
1/4 tsp ground white pepper
1/4 tsp ground ginger
1 bay leaf
2 TBSP grated parmesan cheese

Directions

1. In a large skillet, heat oil. Sauté vermicelli and onion (or celery) until golden brown, about 2 to 4 minutes over medium-high heat. Drain off oil.
2. Add rice, stock, water, pepper, ginger, and bay leaf. Cover and simmer 15-20 minutes.
3. Fluff with fork. Cover and let stand 5-20 minutes. Remove bay leaf.
4. Sprinkle with cheese and serve immediately.

Nutritional information (per serving): Calories 172, Sodium 193mg

*Omit onion in this recipe if it triggers GERD symptoms.

Exotic Asian rice

This recipe uses a variety of ingredients, including pecans and water chestnuts, to make this a unique side dish for any meal. We skim the fat off the chicken stock, skip the salt, and use just a small amount of oil to keep the recipe GERD diet friendly and low in both sodium and fat. We also use a very small amount of fresh onion, but if cooked onion triggers your heartburn symptoms, substitute it with an equivalent amount of dried onion, or omit them from the recipe. Green pepper, celery and long grain rice, seasoned with sage and nutmeg complete the dish! Mmm Mmm, you will savor the exotic flavor!

Recipe makes 10 1/2 cup servings

Ingredients

1 1/2 cup water
1 cup chicken stock or broth, skim fat from top
1 1/3 cup uncooked long-grain white rice
2 tsp vegetable oil
2 TBSP finely chopped onion
2 TBSP finely chopped green pepper
1/2 cup chopped pecans
1/4 tsp ground sage
1 cup finely chopped celery
1/2 cup sliced water chestnuts
1/4 tsp nutmeg
Black pepper to taste

Directions

1. Bring water and chicken stock to a boil in a medium saucepan.
2. Skim the fat from the top, add rice, and stir.
3. Cover and simmer 20 minutes.
4. Remove pan from heat. Let stand, covered, for 5 minutes or until all liquid is absorbed.
5. Heat oil in large nonstick skillet. Sauté onion and celery over medium heat 3 minutes.
6. Stir in remaining ingredients, including reserved cooked rice. Fluff with fork before serving.

Nutritional information (per serving): Calories 139, Sodium 86mg

Vegetable Macaroni and Cheese

Macaroni and cheese, the classic 1950s comfort food, has made a big comeback at restaurants around the country. Once found mostly in diners, "Mac and cheese" has made its way into fine dining establishments and is now even popularly paired with (of all things!) lobster. Though we use vegetables instead of lobster in our GERD-friendly version, you can certainly have some steamed lobster on the side! This recipe uses whole wheat macaroni mixed with chopped cauliflower (or celery), egg whites, and delicious low-fat sharp cheddar cheese. Perfect as a main course or side dish, it takes just minutes to prepare. Then place it in the oven and cook until light golden brown and bubbly! Enjoy!

Makes 4 one cup servings

Ingredients

2 cups whole wheat macaroni
1/2 cup chopped cauliflower
1/2 cup evaporated skim milk
2 egg whites or 1 egg
1/4 tsp ginger
1/4 tsp pepper
1 1/4 cups low fat sharp cheddar cheese
1/2 tsp dried chopped onion seasoning (optional)

Directions

1. Preheat oven to 350 degrees.
2. Cook macaroni according to package directions.
3. Steam or microwave chopped cauliflower and drain well.
4. Place the cauliflower in a large bowl, add the macaroni and remaining ingredients. Mix thoroughly and sprinkle with minced onion, if desired.
5. Transfer the mixture to a casserole dish sprayed with non-stick cooking spray.
6. Place the dish in the oven and bake until bubbly (about 30 minutes).

Nutritional Information: Calories 380, Sodium 120mg

Mini lasagna cups

I am sure you are thinking there is no way lasagna is GERD friendly, right? Well, we make smart modifications to avoid common trigger foods and lighten up a traditionally high fat (and difficult to digest) treat. First, this recipe uses basil pesto instead of tomato sauce. You can make your own pesto or buy pre-made pesto. To reduce the total amount of fat and increase the amount of protein in this dish, we use cottage cheese instead of ricotta and ground turkey instead of ground beef. The pesto sauce contains fat, but it is healthy fat, and pesto is full of vitamins and minerals from the herbs, as well as calcium and vitamin D from the cheese. If you are a vegetarian, try substituting sautéed, chopped mushrooms for the ground turkey.

Recipe serves 12

Ingredients

6 oz. (about 1/3 pound) ground turkey
1 cup low or non–fat cottage cheese
1 ½ cups part skim mozzarella cheese
1 ½ cups shredded parmesan cheese
1 cup pesto sauce (basil & parsley blend)
24 wonton wrappers

Directions

1. Preheat oven to 375 degrees.
2. Prepare a muffin tin by spraying each of the 12 openings with a canola or olive oil spray.
3. Brown the ground turkey in a skillet. Add salt and pepper to taste.
4. Place a wonton wrapper in each muffin cup, and push down into the muffin cups.
5. In each cup, layer the three cheeses, then the meat, then pesto.
6. Place another wonton wrapper on top and repeat layering.
7. Top with the remaining mozzarella and parmesan cheese.
8. Bake for 15-20 minutes until the cheese is melted and the wonton wrappers are browned.
9. Carefully remove from muffin tin and cool before serving.
10. A basil leaf or Kalamata olive (with pit removed) makes a nice garnish!

Nutritional information (per serving): Calories 197, Sodium 400mg

Stuffed Mushroom Caps

Here is a savory recipe that you can bring to a party knowing that your friends won't think you are crazy for trying to bring something healthy. And it's not veggies and dip – usually the default "healthy item" on the buffet table. You can still be original, get your Vitamins D, A, E and many of the B's AND keep your GERD at bay. You can make this vegetarian by leaving out the turkey bacon, but bacon is always a crowd pleaser!

Recipe Serves 6-10 (you can double or triple recipe as needed)

Ingredients

2 cloves Garlic
½ cup Breadcrumbs
6 Slices Turkey Bacon, cooked crispy and crumbled
5 oz Spinach chopped
¼ cups Gruyere - grated
¼ cups Romano – grated
24 medium sized mushrooms, white or brown stems removed (Save the stems to chop and mix with other ingredients)
¼ C olive oil

Directions

1. Preheat oven to 375 degrees.
2. Bake mushroom caps on a greased cookie sheet tops facing up for about 10 minutes.
3. Chop garlic, mushroom stems, and turkey bacon. Saute in olive oil over medium heat until all are tender and beginning to brown (about 5 minutes).
4. Add spinach and continue sautéing for 3 minutes more until spinach is wilted.
5. In a large bowl mix, breadcrumbs and cheese. Once stove mixture is finished, add it to the bowl with breadcrumbs and cheese. Combine thoroughly.
6. Fill the mushroom caps with mixture.
7. Place on baking sheet a second time and bake again for 10-15 more minutes.

Nutritional Information (Per Serving): Calories 105, Sodium 800mg

Cantaloupe sorbet

This icy cold sorbet is so refreshing. It has a creamy, full-bodied flavor with a light, smooth texture. The recipe contains only three ingredients, so it's incredibly easy to throw together. Just be sure to chill the melons well in the hours before, so that the sorbet will freeze up even faster. Cantaloupes are packed with healthy nutrients and are a safe fruit for people who need to keep a GERD friendly diet. It's a palate-cleansing sweet finale to an evening meal!

Makes about 6 servings

Ingredients
1 cup sugar
1 cup water
4 cups cantaloupe, chilled

Directions
1. Place the water and sugar in a small saucepan and bring to a boil, stirring constantly to dissolve the sugar to make a syrup.
2. Remove from heat and place in an airtight container. Place in freezer until cold (about 2 hours).
3. Peel, seed, and cube cantaloupe and keep chilled.
4. Combine the cold syrup with the chilled cantaloupe in a large mixing bowl, and blend until fluffy using an electric mixer.
5. Return to freezer and freeze overnight until firm.

Nutritional information (per serving): Calories 116, Sodium 15mg

Pineapple ambrosia

"Ambrosia" is a family favorite, and this recipe is a lightened up GERD diet friendly version. Ambrosia is a variation on the traditional fruit salad, which typically contains oranges, a common GERD trigger, so we substituted fresh peaches, which worked well. Be sure when selecting a peach to look for an even color, and the flesh should have a slight give. We combined sugar-free pudding with reduced-calorie whipped topping and folded in a healthy trio of peach, banana, and pineapple. And last but not least, the crushed graham crackers add the perfect crunch and sweetness to this after dinner treat! Enjoy!

Yields 6 servings

Ingredients
1 package sugar-free instant vanilla pudding mix (4 serving)
1 cup nonfat dry milk powder
1 1/2 cups water
2 TBSP white vinegar
4 white peaches (medium ripe)
1 (8 ounce) can crushed pineapple, undrained
1 cup reduced-calorie whipped topping
1 cup diced banana
9 (2-1/2 inch) graham crackers (coarsely crushed)

Directions
1. Mix dry milk powder, water, and vinegar in a large bowl and let set for 6 minutes.
2. Add undrained pineapple and pudding mix to the bowl. Mix with a wire whisk until well blended.
3. Stir in whipped topping.
4. Chop the peaches into one inch bites, and add them to the mixture.
5. Add the diced banana and crushed graham crackers, reserving 3 tablespoons for topping.
6. Blend well and evenly spoon into 6 dessert dishes.
7. Sprinkle remaining crumbs over the top of each dish, and refrigerate for at least 15 minutes.

Nutritional information (per serving): Calories 165, Sodium 238mg

Vanilla almond parfait

This cold dessert recipe is made the day before and chilled overnight in the refrigerator. It is made with layers of fruit and yogurt and contains nutrient packed chia seeds. The word "chia" means "strength" and the fruit is a popular energy food choice for athletes and hikers. The chia seeds are tiny and easy to add to a wide variety of dishes, including desserts. We use agave, a "natural sweetener, to keep this tasty parfait lower in calories. Its healthy ingredients make it guilt free and GERD diet friendly, so enjoy!

Makes 4 servings

Ingredients

1 cup vanilla almond milk (unsweetened)
1 cup Greek yogurt (plain low fat)
2 TBSP agave
1 tsp vanilla
1/8 tsp kosher salt
1/4 cup chia seeds
2 cups sliced strawberries
1/4 cup sliced almonds
4 tsp agave for serving

Directions

1. Place the first five ingredients in a medium bowl and whisk gently until well blended.
2. Blend in the chia seeds and let sit for 25 minutes.
3. Stir, cover, and refrigerate overnight.
4. When ready to serve, toss the strawberries with the remaining 4 tsp agave and mix in the toasted almonds.
5. Make layers of the pudding and berry mixture in glass parfait dishes or sturdy glasses.

Nutritional information (per serving): Calories 199, Sodium 197mg

Baked bananas

This simple recipe is delicious and a delightful treat for breakfast or dessert. Bananas are naturally sweet, rich in healthy potassium, and are considered a safe fruit for people who have acid reflux. Other ingredients, including coconut, ginger, and cinnamon, are GERD diet friendly. For breakfast, I serve the bananas alone or with oatmeal on the side - or topped with chopped nuts or raisins if I have them on hand. For an after dinner treat, I enjoy them with a scoop of frozen yogurt! Mmm mmm good!

Serves 6

Ingredients

6 large bananas, ripe but still firm
2 TBSP low fat margarine
2 tsp cinnamon
2 tsp ginger
1/4 cup apple juice
3 Tablespoons shredded coconut
Low fat frozen yogurt
Nuts and raisins

Directions

1. Preheat oven to 350 degrees.
2. Peel bananas and brush each with melted low fat margarine.
3. Sprinkle each banana with a small amount of freshly ground ginger and apple juice.
4. Top with shredded coconut and cinnamon.
5. Place bananas in a shallow baking dish.
6. Bake in a 350 degree oven for 20 minutes.
7. Serve alone or with a side of frozen yogurt.

Nutritional information (per banana): Calories 190, Sodium 44mg

Peachy cobbler

This dessert recipe is made with heartburn friendly fruits and juices and flavored up with nutmeg and cinnamon, which are GERD diet friendly spices. We kept the dish low in fat by using evaporated skim milk and cooking oil spray to coat the pan. You'll be surprised how quick and easy it is to make, so give it a try. It's perfect for any occasion!

Makes 8 servings

Ingredients

1/2 tsp ground cinnamon
1 TBSP vanilla extract
2 TBSP cornstarch
1 cup peach nectar
1/4 cup pineapple juice or peach juice
2 16-oz cans peaches, sliced, packed in juice, drained (or 1-3/4 lbs fresh)
1 TBSP margarine
1 cup dry pancake mix
2/3 cup all-purpose flour
1/2 cup sugar
2/3 cup evaporated skim milk
Nonstick cooking oil spray (for baking dish)
Topping: 1/2 tsp nutmeg and 1 TBSP brown sugar

Directions

1. Combine cinnamon, vanilla, cornstarch, peach nectar, and pineapple or peach juice in a saucepan over medium heat. Stir constantly until mixture thickens and bubbles.
2. Add sliced peaches to mixture.
3. Reduce heat and simmer for 5 to 10 minutes.
4. In another saucepan melt margarine and set aside.
5. Lightly spray an 8-inch square glass dish with cooking oil spray. Pour hot peach mixture into the dish.
6. In another bowl, combine pancake mix, flour, sugar, and melted margarine. Stir in milk.
7. Quickly spoon this mixture over peach mixture.
8. Combine nutmeg and brown sugar. Sprinkle mixture on top of batter.
9. Bake at 400 degrees F for 15 to 20 minutes or until golden brown.
10. Cool and cut into 8 squares.

Nutritional information (per serving): Calories 271, Sodium 263mg

Banana Date Mousse

This healthy mousse will safely and surely satisfy your sweet tooth! It is a perfect light dessert recipe, and it's quick and easy to prepare in your blender. We recommend using ripe bananas and Medjool dates, which are non-acidic fruits that are easy on the stomach and GERD friendly! If you have never tried dates, they are a real treat and one of my favorite natural sweeteners. Like bananas, dates contain lots of vitamins and minerals that promote good health. We use raw sugar in this recipe, but you may prefer a sugar substitute. Enjoy!

Serves 4

Ingredients
2 T low fat milk
4 tsp raw sugar or sugar substitute*
1 tsp vanilla
1 medium ripe banana, cut in quarters
1 cup plain low-fat yogurt
8 1/4 inch banana slices
2 to 3 ounces coarsely chopped Medjool dates

Directions
1. Place milk, sugar, vanilla, and banana in blender.
2. Process 15 seconds at high speed until smooth.
3. Pour mixture into a small bowl.
4. Fold in yogurt.
5. Chill well in the refrigerator for at least one hour.
6. Spoon into four dessert dishes. Top with banana slices and chopped dates just before serving.

Nutritional information (per serving): Calories 145, Sodium 48mg

*Be sure to check package labels on sweeteners for adjusted amount recommendation.

Coconut rice pudding

Coconuts contain natural sugar and can be a delicious and healthy way to add some sweetness to your diet. There are no "trigger" ingredients in this recipe and we have noticed frequent discussion on the Internet about coconut being helpful to GERD sufferers - you will have to be the judge! This recipe is quick and easy and a twist on an all-time favorite dessert. But for those watching their cholesterol, keep in mind that coconut milk contains some saturated fat so this recipe might not be the right choice for you.

Makes about 6 servings

Ingredients

3/4 cup low-fat milk
1/2 cup coconut milk
1 large pear grated
2 TBPS honey
1 (1oz) package instant fat-free, sugar-free vanilla pudding mix
2 cups cooked rice
1/4 cup shredded coconut
1/2 tsp ground ginger

Directions

1. Bring the first four listed ingredients to a boil over medium heat and immediately remove from heat.
2. Slowly mix in pudding with a wire whisk.
3. Stir in rice, coconut, and ginger.
4. Let mixture sit for 10 minutes to blend flavors, stirring occasionally.
5. Top with berries if desired. Can be served warm or cold.

Nutritional information (per serving): Calories 190, Sodium 244mg

Strawberry cream with mango and honey sauce

This is a smooth and luscious, yet very healthy dessert. We use strawberries in this creamy delight, but you can substitute raspberries, blueberries, kiwi, pineapple chunks, or even bananas. All of these fruits have an abundance of health benefits and are GERD diet friendly, so you can use whatever you have on hand for convenience. We also recommend that you use "local" honey for good health, because it contains pollen from your local area, which helps to strengthen and build up your immunities. This is an after dinner treat recipe that's easy to make and sure to become one of your family favorites!

Yields 4 servings

Ingredients

1/2 cup low fat cream cheese
1/2 cup Greek yogurt
2 TBSP confectioners sugar
1 large ripe mango
1 TBSP honey
1 cup sliced strawberries

Directions

1. Soften the cream cheese and mix well with the sugar and yogurt.
2. Peel the flesh off the mango and cut into small chunks.
3. Purée mango in a blender or food processor. Add honey to the purée by first dipping a tablespoon into boiling water, wipe the spoon dry, and then the honey should easily slide off the spoon. Blend briefly.
4. Evenly divide the strawberries (reserving 4 or 8 slices) into four dessert glasses.
5. Top the strawberries with the evenly divided cream cheese yogurt mixture (reserving 4 TBSP). Smooth the cream cheese mixture down nicely.
6. Cover with the mango purée and top each with a reserved TBSP of cream cheese and 1 or 2 reserved strawberries slices.

Nutritional information (per serving): Calories 165, Sodium 35mg

Peanut butter milkshake

Peanut butter and bananas are a popular duo, so it's not surprising that the combination makes a tasty milk shake. Blend these two great flavors together along with a few other ingredients, and you will feel like you just made a trip to an ice cream shop. It's a lightened-up GERD-diet friendly treat that you can make in just seconds!

Yields 2 servings

Ingredients
1-1/2 cups skim milk
1 large ripe banana (chilled in freezer or refrigerator)
2 TBSP reduced fat peanut butter
1/2 cup frozen vanilla ice cream (sugar and fat free)
1 tsp honey

Directions
1. Combine bananas and milk in a blender.
2. Cover and blend for 25 seconds.
3. Add peanut butter, ice cream and honey and blend until smooth about 20 more seconds.
4. Serve immediately.

Nutritional information (per serving): Calories 274, Sodium 211mg

Appendices

Food Calorie Chart

This food chart is taken from the CalorieKing Food and Nutrition Database (www.calorieking.com), product labels, and from specific company websites. Parenthesis indicates a specific company product or brand.

Food Item	Quantity	CAL	SOD	Food Group
Almonds (.3 cup)	1.0 oz.	164	0	1.0 nuts/seeds
Apple	1.0 medium	92	3	1.0 fruit
Apple	1.0 large 120	3		1.0 fruit
Apple Juice	1.0 cup	120	10	2.0 fruit
Asparagus	1.0 cup	40	25	2.0 vegetables
Avocado	2.0 oz.	95	5	0.5 fruit
Bagel	1.0 mini 72	139		1.0 grain
Bagel - cinnamon raisin	1.0 medium	287	338	2.0 grain
Bagel - whole wheat	1.0 large 300	470		2.0 grain
Banana	1.0 medium	105	1	1.0 fruit
Blueberries - frozen/raw	0.3 cup	24	0	1.0 fruit
Beef - eye round	0.3 oz.	109	20	4.0 meat/fish/poultry
Beef - filet mignon	3.0 oz.	153	54	3.0 meat/fish/poultry
Beef - frankfurter- 5"	1.0 link	165	570	2.0 meat/fish/poultry
Beef - ground 95% lean	3.0 oz.	111	49	3.0 meat/fish/poultry
Beef - pastrami	4.0 oz.	41	251	4.0 meat/fish/poultry
Beef - sirloin (broiled)	3.0 oz.	100	35	3.0 meat/fish/poultry
Beef - T-bone (broiled)	4.0 oz.	200	80	4.0 meat/fish/poultry
Beans, green	0.5 cup	22	1	1.0 vegetable
Beans, edamame (raw)	10.0 pods	29	3	0.5 vegetables
Beans, refried, canned	0.5 cup	118	377	1.0 Nuts/Seeds/Legumes
Bread - White	1.0 slice	24	44	1.0 grain
Bread - Whole Wheat (Safeway)	1.0 slice	90	150	1.0 grain
Bread - Rye	1.0 slice	18	46	1.0 grain
Broccoli - steamed	1.0 cup	55	64	2.0 vegetables
Brussels Sprouts - boiled	0.5 cup	28	16	1.0 vegetables
Butter - Unsalted	1.0 tsp	34	1	1.0 fats/oils
Cabbage, boiled	1.0 cup	33	12	2.0 vegetables
Cantaloupe	1.0 cup	53	13	2.0 fruit
Carrots - shredded	0.3 cups	14	23	0.5 vegetable
Carrots - sliced	0.5 cups	25	42	1.0 vegetable
Cashews, dry roasted no salt	1.0 tbsp	49	1	0.5 nuts/seeds
Cauliflower	0.5 cup	13	16	1.0 vegetable
Celery - raw (7 inch)	1.0 stalk	6	32	1.0 vegetable

Cheese - Blue	1.0 oz.	100	395	1.0 dairy
Cheese - Cheddar/Colby low fat	1.0 oz.	29	104	1.0 dairy
Cheese - Laughing Cow	2.0 wedges	100	420	2.0 dairy
Cheese - Provolone low fat	1.0 slice	77	245	0.75 dairy
Cheese, Romano grated	1.0 tbsp	20	85	0.2 dairy
Cheese, string - Lite Sargento	2.0 Pcs	120	220	1.5 dairy
Cheese, swiss	1.0 oz.	108	54	1.0 dairy
Cheese, swiss low fat	1.0 oz.	51	74	1.0 dairy
Chex mix - standard mix	1.0 cup	240	420	2.0 grain
Chicken Breast Meat	3.0 oz.	140	63	3.0 meat/fish/poultry
Celery - chopped	1.0 tbsp	4	23	N/A
Cereal - Raisin Bran (Kellogg)	1.0 cup	190	210	2.0 grains
Cereal - Cheerios	1.0 cup	100	160	1.0 grains
Cereal - corn flakes	1.0 cup.	113	199	1.0 grains
Cereal - Frosted Flakes (Kellogg)	1.0 cup	147	200	1.5 grains
Cereal - Frosted Wheat (Fiber One)	1.0 cup	200	0	2.0 grains
Cereal - Granola (Open Nature)	0.5 cup	280	110	1.5 grains
Cereal - Granola, Oats, Honey Almonds (Quaker)	1.0 cup	400	50	3.0 grains
Cereal - Lucky Charms	1.0 cup	147	227	1.5 grains
Cereal - Total (General Mills)	1.0 cup	133	253	1.5 grains
Coconut - shredded	0.5 cup	233	122	1.0 fruit
Cookie - oatmeal raisin	1 cookie	200	130	1.0 sweet
Cookie - double chocolate chip	1 cookie	210	130	1.0 sweet
Corn - Canned Yellow Sweet	1.0 cup	133	351	2.0 vegetables
Corn - White, sweet on cob	1.0 ear	59	3	1.0 vegetables
Cottage Cheese 2%	0.5 cup	102	460	1.0 dairy
Crackers - Wheat Thins (Nabisco)	10.0 pcs	88	144	1.0 grain
Crackers - Whole Wheat	6.0 Pcs	84	144	1.0 grain
Cranberries - Jellied (Ocean Spray)	1.0 tbsp	28	3	.25 fruit
Cream Cheese - Low fat.	1.0 tbsp	23	30	0.3 dairy
Cucumber - Sliced	0.5 cups	8	1	1.0 vegetable
Dressing - Ranch Fat Free	1.0 tbsp	13	180	0.5 fats/oils
Egg - Hardboiled	1.0 large	78	62	1.0 dairy
Egg Substitute - Eggbeaters	0.25 cup	30	115	1.0 meat/fish/poultry
English Muffin - Cinn/Raisin	1.0 medium	140	170	2.0 grain
English Muffin - Whole Wheat	1.0 medium	120	220	2.0 grain
Fruit Cocktail	1.0 cup	109	9	2.0 fruit
Fruit - Mixed and Dried	0.3 cups	138	10	1.0 fruit
Garbanzo beans	1.0 cup	269	80	2.0 nuts/seeds

Graham Crackers	2 large	118	169	1.0 grain
Grits, white corn	0.5 cup	71	2	1.0 grain
Grape Juice	1.0 cup	170	20	2.0 fruit
Grapes - red or green	1.0 cup	104	3	2.0 fruit
Gravy - brown/dry pkg	1.0 tbsp	22	291	N/A
Granola Bar - (Quaker Nut Chewy)	1.0 bar	140	65	1.0 nuts/seeds
Green Beans - fresh / boiled	1.0cup	40	0	2.0 vegetables
Halibut - baked	4.0 oz.	159	78	4.0 meat/fish/poultry
Hamburger Bun - Whole Wheat	1.0 large	120	150	2.0 grains
Ham	1.0 oz	46	375	1.0 meat/fish/poultry
Honey	1.0tbsp	64	1	N/A
Hummus - Roast Red Pepper	2.0 tbsp	70	120	1.0 nuts/seeds
Hummus - Greek Olive (Sabra)	2.0 tbsp	70	130	1.0 nuts/seeds
Jam/Jelly - (Smucker's)	1.0 tbsp	50	0	N/A
Jell-O (Spangles)	6.0 oz.	15	83	N/A
Kale, raw	1.0 cup	34	29	2.0 vegetables
Lettuce - butterhead	0.3 cup	2	1	0.5 vegetable
Lettuce - Iceberg Shredded	0.3 cups	2	2	0.5 vegetable
Lettuce - Romaine	1.0 leaf	1	0	0.3 vegetable
Margarine - soft	1.0 tsp	33	31	1.0 fats/oils
Margarine - (Smart Balance)	1.0 tbsp	80	90	3.0 fats/oils
Mayonnaise - reduced fat	1.0 tbsp	49	101	N/A
Milk - Coconut	0.5 cup	90	24	1.0 fruit
Milk - Fat Free Skim	1.0 cups	90	125	1.0 dairy
Mushrooms - fresh sliced	1.0 oz.	6	1	0.5 vegetable
Mushrooms - Portabella	1.0 oz.	6	3	0.5 vegetables
Mustard - Dijon	1.0 tsp	5	120	N/A
Oatmeal - instant regular	0.5 cup	83	5	1.0 grain
Olives - green, pitted	0.5 cup	25	115	N/A
Pasta - whole wheat	0.5 cup	87	1	1 grain
Peaches	0.5 cup	52	5	1 fruit
Peach Nectar	1.0 cup	134	17	2 fruits
Pear	1.0 small	84	1	1.0 fruit
Peanut butter.	1.0 tbsp	85	70.	0.5 nut
Peas - boiled w/o salt	0.5 cup	125	38	1.0 vegetable
Peas and carrots w/o salt	0.5 cup	48	5	1.0 vegetable
Pineapple	2.0 slices	56	1	1 fruit
Pineapple juice	1.0 cup	133	5	2 fruit
Pita Bread - Wheat	1.0 reg	90	320	2.0 grain
Pita chips - Stacy's Cinn/Sug	7.0 chips	140	115	1.0 grain

Popcorn - (Redenbacker Smartpop)	1.0 minibag	100	150	1 vegetable
Potato - Baked	1.0 medium	168	14	2.0 vegetable
Potato - Baked	1.0 large	278	30	2.5 vegetables
Potato - Red (4" diam)	1.0 large	266	24	2.0 vegetables
Potato - Sweet / baked	1.0 large	16	6	2.0 vegetable
Pretzels - unsalted sourdough (Snyder's)	20 mini	110	75	2.0 grains
Raisins - seedless	0.3 cup	130	5	1.0 fruit
Raisins - seedless	1.0 oz.	85	3	0,5 fruit
Pudding - Vanilla Sugar Free	0.5 cup	64	193	N/A
Rice - Brown/Long Grain	0.5 cups	108	5	1.0 grain
Rice - White/Medium Grain	0.5 cups	121	0	1.0 grain
Rice - Wild	0.5 cup	83	2	1.0 grain
Roll - Whole Wheat Dinner	1.0 small	74	147	1.0 grain
Roll - Standard dinner	1.0 small	87	150	1.0 grain
Shrimp	3.0 oz.	84	191	3.0 meat/fish/poultry
Sorbet - Coconut (Whole Fruit)	0.5 cup	150	10	N/A
Sour Cream - low fat	1.0 tbsp	16	9	0.75 dairy
Spinach - Raw	1.0 cup	7	24	2.0 vegetable
Spinach - frozen.	1.0 cup	27	227	2.0 vegetable
Strawberries	0.5 cup	24	1	1.0 fruit
Sweet Potato - baked	0.5 large	80	32	1.0 vegetable
Sweet Potato - Fries (Ore-Ida)	3 oz.	160	160	1.0 vegetable
Tartar Sauce	1.0 tsp	18	33	N/A
Tilapia - Steamed	0.4 oz.	146	63	4.0 meat/fish/poultry
Tortilla - White Corn	1.0 unit	45	0	1.0 grain
Triscuits Whole Grain	6.0 Pcs	103	137	1.0 grain
Triscuits - Brown Rice	6.0 Pcs	87	73	1.0 grain
Tuna - light in water	2.0 oz.	66	192	2.0 meat/fish/poultry
Turkey - (Columbus Brand) Low sodium slices	2.0 oz.	60	230	2.0 meat/fish/poultry
Turkey Burger - jenny O	3.0 oz.	137	76	3.0 meat/fish/poultry
Vegetable burger - Boca	2.5 oz.	80	300	1.0 vegetable
Walnuts	1.0 oz.	185	1	1.0 nuts
Yogurt - Low-fat Fruit	6.0 oz.	174	99	0.5 dairy
Yogurt - No fat - plain (Chobani)	5.3 oz.	90	70	0.5 dairy
Yogurt - Frozen	0.5 cup	80	80	0.5 dairy
Yogurt - Frozen Strawberry (Yogurt Land)	0.5 cup	110	60	0.5 dairy
Yogurt - Frozen Vanilla, Greek Low fat (Yoplait)	0.5 cup	110	80	0.5 dairy

Made in the USA
Middletown, DE
20 November 2017